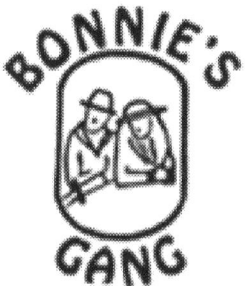

Bonnie's Gang Publishing is proud to present:

The fourth in a series of works for lovers.
Also by Jani:

The G-gasm Method

Tonight's the Night: Ultimate Guide to Sexy, Kinky Things to do With Your Lover

BlowPons … Blowjob Coupons

The G-Gasm Method For Lesbian Lovers

*Your Ultimate Guide to the G-spot Orgasm
How to Have Your Woman Experience 10, 20 or Even 50 Big O's Per Night.*

G-gasm Method for Lesbian Lovers:
Your Ultimate Guide to the G-spot Orgasm
How to Have Your Woman Experience
10, 20 or Even 50 Big O's Per Night.

By: Jani - Published by Bonnie's Gang Publishing, New York

Although based on actual experience, some events in this book have been fictionalized to protect the privacy of certain individuals.

Please consult your Doctor if you are pregnant, have had a caesarean, surgery or infections before trying the G-gasm Method. As with anything, use common sense.

Copyright 2007 Bonnie's Gang

All rights reserved. No part of this book may be reproduced, stored in a retrieval system, transmitted in electronic form, or any other means reproduced without the prior permission of Bonnie's Gang.

Bonnie's Gang Publishing

Please visit us at:
G-gasm.com

ISBN # 0-9762090-6-3

With thanks for pioneering the G-spot to

Dr. Gräfenberg

CONTENTS

Preface - 11

Introduction to G-spot Orgasms - 15

Getting Started - 21 – What is a G-gasm – 22 What and Where is the G-spot? – 23

The G-gasm Method – 29 No Sex Toy Needed – 32 Rules – 35 Cunnilingus and the G-gasm Method – 39 The Next Level – 44 Female Ejaculation / Squirting – 45 Squirting Guidelines – 48 PC Muscles / Kegel Exercises - 49

Variations of the G-gasm Method – Page 52 You Are In Control – 53 BDSM Fun – You Are So Naughty – 58 Edging: What Is It and How – 64 Working the G-gasm Method - 73

Multiple Vaginal Orgasms – The Best Part – Page 78 Strap-On Sex - 78 Strap on With Jena – 79 G-gasms Feel Like … - 81

Email … We get email – Page – 83

AutoGasms – 95

Warning … Extremely Powerful – Page 97 Appendix - 101

PREFACE

Having good sex isn't like mathematics where what you punch into a calculator is either right or wrong – sex is much more complicated than that. The only way you know if you are performing well is by the reactions of your partner.

Years ago while struggling through college, I was in a committed relationship with a fellow student, since I was at best an ordinary learner, it was the high point of my years there. Years later, I looked back on that relationship and winced. Our sex life was so bad – we did not have a clue how to please each other.

After college, I worked as a bartender in various nice restaurants and gin mills – that was my real higher learning center for life. I like having those relationships as memories but I would be embarrassed to have anyone else know about them.

It is not as if I frown when thinking back about my lack of knowledge and experience about sex, what concerned me more was – when and how do I get good.

I found most of the lesbian books to be on target, but missed the mark on one very important issue. I resurrected and studied Dr. Gräfenberg work, which the G-spot is named after, and came to a hypothesis about repeating

G-spot orgasms.

What followed was a series of hands on experiments, in other words taking what Dr. Gräfenberg put on paper to studying on actual ladies and how they react to G-spot manipulation

I did not test on cadavers, instead all testing done in a "hands on" manner. With all due respect to Doctors and their profession, sometimes I think these so called experts do not test their theories on a real life girlfriend.

This book has boundaries otherwise it would be volumes. This book isn't an encyclopedia, a psychoanalytical book or an anthology. If you are looking for technical data or biological information about the vagina then you should look elsewhere. Looking for information about how the brain influences orgasms? It's not here. Anthology of lesbian sex stories? Nope.

I've set out to write a thorough book about G-spot stimulation and within the boundaries of that form, I can go to work.

I hope your sex life improves tonight – enjoy.

INTRODUCTION TO G-SPOT ORGASMS

> "Pulling my sweetheart close to me, her hips reacting to the gentle tug ... my hand reaches up towards her soft shoulders, her head tilts ... my moist lips caress the skin under her ear ... she nudges me on ... I softly bite the area that joins her neck and shoulder, she places her hands around my shoulders ... our lips meet ..."

Before my current long-term relationship, I had more than my share of girlfriends. I was in my mid 20's and during this period, all I was looking for in relationships were FWBs or "friends with benefits." I had no interest in any kind of long-term relationship. I just wanted to have some fun and move on to the next woman. During this time, I met a FWB named Nikki.

Nikki was in her early 30's and even more of a horn-dog than I was. We understood each other perfectly. Neither one of us was looking for commitment. We could be open and honest, and often discussed our sexual conquests. It did not take long before we ratcheted our friendship up a notch. If either one of us had a blank spot on our dating card, we knew who to call. Nikki was the most responsive woman I had ever met. Her clit was like a detonator switch. One touch with my tongue and she would explode. It was like fireworks; beautiful to watch but never lasted long enough.

Nikki had been away, and I had been yearning for her while she was on her trip. As a little something special, I wanted to let her know she was missed and how glad I was to have her back.

I invited Nikki to come over to my place for the evening. I was not a great cook by any means, but I could order out with the best of them. Everything was ready. I lit the candles, had a bottle of white wine on ice, some John Coltrane playing; the mood was set for some serious loving. Body oil, lube and a couple of vibrators crammed the bedside table drawer.

Before Nikki had left on her trip we had talked about G-spots, and while she was away, I had read about and learned the secrets of mastering the G-spot. I had an idea - The G-gasm Method - and I wanted to share it with her.

To say Nikki was hot was an understatement. She was not classically beautiful, but she did not have to be. She was confident and completely at ease with her body. The sexual vibe rolled off her, and when she walked down the street, heads tuned so fast I swear some of those people surely got whiplash. I felt especially sorry for the guys, knowing they didn't have a chance. Nikki combed her fingers through that long brown hair and worked those hips in a way that made every butch within a mile take notice. And when she wore high heels ... Ok, so maybe I have a little bit of a foot fetish, but the shoes made her smoking hot.

Nikki arrived at my place around seven o'clock. I gently kissed her warm perfumed skin and thought of how beautiful she looked when I opened the door to greet her.

Her black shirt stretched across her chest, contrasting sharply with her smooth soft milky white skin. It was obvious that she was not wearing a bra because her nipples were clearly visible beneath the fabric. I wanted to touch them so badly, but I made myself wait.

My arms encircled her as I leaned towards her and she raised her head to meet my waiting lips. Kissing her softly at first, I then nibbled on her bottom lips before taking it between my teeth and sucking. With my tongue, I explored her mouth insistently, yet gently. My hands slowly slid down her back until they rested on Nikki's wonderful ass. She raised her head and smiled at me, and I knew then that she wanted me as much as I wanted her.

As I poured her a glass of wine, Nikki stepped up from behind, and wrapped her arms around my waist. Her wandering hands trailed down past my belt buckle and teasingly tugged on the strap-on I was wearing.

"Feels like you prepared for anything," Nikki breathed against the back of my neck.

"I aim to please, ma'am," I said in my best imitation of a western drawl. We both laughed, not because it was funny but to ease some of the built-up tension. Taking the glass from her hand and placing it on the table, I guided her to my bedroom. I sat down on the king size bed and pulled her into my lap. We kissed deeply, while I ran my hands up and down her legs and body. Her emerald green eyes looked deeply into mine, and her face spread into a wicked, naughty grin.

Without breaking eye contact, I pushed her legs apart, ran my hand up the inside of Nikki's thigh and beneath her skirt. Nikki gasped and trembled a bit, as her breath grew shorter. I found the edge of her panties and slid a finger under the elastic, parting her moist curls and slipping between the folds. Nikki bucked hard against my hand, but I teasingly withdrew it and continued to stroke the inside of her thighs. Every now and then, I would go back to her mound but never quite make it inside her panties again. My finger would rub up against her clit through the thin material and she would let out a soft frustrated moan.

She unbuttoned my shirt and ran her long fingers from my collarbone down to the tops of my breasts. Her red polished nails playfully flicked my hard nipples until they were raspberry red. Nikki gave me a seductive glance, slid off my lap and got on her knees between my legs. She knelt there for a minute, running her hands up and down my thighs, getting closer and closer to the dildo I wore.

Smiling, she pressed me back to a reclining position. Her hands ran over my stomach, circling my navel before she bent her head and traced a circle around my bellybutton. Nikki's tongue dipped into the depression there as she unbuckled my belt and opened my jeans. Her tongue was hot on my lower abdomen and as I arched up, she pushed my jeans to the floor.

Nikki leaned in close, and ran her fingers along the leather straps that wrapped around my waist and thighs. She playfully stroked and kissed the base of the dildo, then worked her soft lips and tongue slowly and teasingly up the shaft. She took the head between her lips, and gently rolled her tongue around the rim. On every downward stroke, very slowly, she applied more and more pressure. I felt it all the way from my clit to my toes. Nikki often made me come just by working the dildo in circles against my clit and I sometimes wondered just where she learned that particular talent. But tonight when she took her lips off me for a second to catch her breath, I lifted her to her feet and spun her on the bed next to me. Tonight, I had different plans.

I raised Nikki's blouse over her head and slipped it off, exposing her breasts. Her nipples were dusky pink and as hard as little pebbles. I unzipped her jeans, slipped them down over her ass and threw them to the floor.

I tweaked and teased the nipple of one breast with my fingers as I nibbled the other one tenderly. Meanwhile, my other hand cupped her crotch through her moist panties. I could feel how wet she was getting and the scent of her arousal nearly made me crazy.

We continued kissing, caressing and licking every inch of our bodies that we could reach. We had already played with spanking before, so I tied Nikki's arms and hands to the bedposts with silk ties I had laid out earlier. She was now face down and spread-eagled across the bed. Nikki thought I was going to smack her ass and the thought made her dripping wet with excitement.

I couldn't help smiling when Nikki thought she was about to get some spanking action. I have yet to find another woman who enjoyed a little bondage as much as Nikki did. Now, I am not talking about inflicting pain or anything. That is a completely different topic. What I am talking about is the act of lovingly spanking a beautiful bottom, which Nikki certainly had.

"You haven't spanked me for a long time..." Nikki whispered as she wiggled her butt up in the air.

It was very sexy, having her in that position asking me to spank her. I have a theory, the butt, both nipples and the vagina are all somehow wired together. Touching, squeezing, pinching or kissing any one part causes a reaction in the other two. I have nearly short-circuited a time or two when one of my girlfriends decided to slap my ass during an orgasm.

I gave Nikki a couple of smacks just to get her all warmed up and wanting more. We had been experimenting with a foam backed ping-pong paddle. Nikki was loud - I mean LOUD. She was not shy about vocalizing her pleasure.

I pulled her panties aside and rubbed the dildo up and down and across her pussy, just barely grazing the lips with the head. She tried to shove her ass back toward me, in a vain effort to get some relief.

"I don't think you're ready for me are you," I teased. "I'm not sure you want it badly enough."

Moving over her, I raised one knee between her legs and pressed. She was hot and wet against my skin. I replaced my knee with my fingers, dipping into all that wet heat and stroking.

"Please fuck me - don't make me wait," Nikki whispered.

"Don't worry, you're going to get fucked," I said as I rocked into her. "But I have other plans first."

Nikki nodded meekly as I continued to play with her lips, spreading them apart and fingering her wet hole.

GETTING STARTED

Listen up ladies; you are about to learn a life changing sex method. Sex will never be as it once was - once you master this, she will be your sex slave forever.

This Method is easy to learn, some practice to master. Once you, and the lucky woman you are trying the G-gasm Method on, find the right spot, she will be so happy she will be telling all her girlfriends. Then what are you going to do? You will have girls lining up at your bedroom door.

The G-gasm Method will make you a confident lover. You will make any woman multi orgasmic. You will learn the skills to please any and every woman. It doesn't matter who you are or what kind of person you are, when you try this Method, you will succeed and she will thank you for it. OK, 'thank you' is a very mild way of saying, "THAT WAS FAN-FUCKING-TASTIC!" You are about to learn how to give your lady the ultimate in pleasure and satisfaction.

I am not a celebrity or a sex therapist. I am not a doctor so this book will not provide you with any form of medical jargon. You will not find a flow chart of the vagina or any type of medical advice that you could expect to find when you are speaking to a doctor. If you are looking for that kind of information, I am sorry, Yahoo "woman's vagina" – you will get all the info you need. There is not a doctor in the world that will teach you, what you are about to learn here.

I have never really kept track, but I have made love to over 50 women. I have no medical training but I can teach you plenty of things about a woman's body, her G-spot and the right way to stimulate it to create orgasm after mind blowing orgasm. The G-gasm Method is not hard to do once you know exactly where to find the G-spot, and how to fire it up correctly.

Reading this, means you are curious about pleasing a woman in a new way. You can make it happen; this method works. I am offering you the guidance and knowledge needed to perform this Method. In time, your girlfriend / lover / FWB will believe you are a superstar in the bedroom.

WHAT IS A G-GASM?

LET US FIRST DEFINE ORGASM.

The meaning of life.

A discharge of neuromuscular tensions at the apex of sexual stimulation that is accompanied by the ejaculation of semen in men and by vaginal contractions and possibly a "squirt" in the female.

An explosion inside your body.

The best possible feeling … ever.

OOOOh yes! Yes! AHHH! Baby yes Baby yes yes! OOOoooh ooooh ooooh OOOH! Harder baby! Yes! Yes! YES! YES!!! Yes! YES! YES! Oh yeah! Your make me so fuckin' horny! Yes!

Take your pick. One or more of the preceding is the correct definition of "orgasm."

Direct G-spot stimulation produces waves of G-gasms. There are plenty of "doctors" that will swear there is no such thing as a "vaginal orgasm." These same experts will tell you that the only way to achieve female orgasm is by direct stimulation of the clitoris. Recent discoveries about the size of the clitoris - it extends inside the body - would seem to support my theory about G-gasms. The nerves of the clitoris pass through the G-spot and connect to the spinal cord for transmission to the brain cells. As the G-spot is stimulated, it grows in size. How awesome is that?

You are about to learn how to "wake up" the G-spot and make it explode. The method for G-spot stimulation you are about to learn will produce G-gasm after G-gasm. Again, a G-gasm is an orgasm achieved through direct stimulation of the G-spot not from the stimulation of the clitoris.

WHAT AND WHERE IS THE G-SPOT?

Back in 1950 there was a doctor Ernest Gräfenberg, M.D., who wrote the now famous article "The Role of Urethra in Female Orgasm." The article gets a little technical, but here are some excerpts of the important points that are relevant to G-gasms.

"A rather high percentage of women do not reach the climax in sexual intercourse. The frigidity figures of different authors vary from 10-80 per cent and come closer to the statistics of older sexologists. Adler (Berlin) concluded that 80 per cent of women did not reach the sexual climax. Moosean guessed that 50 per cent suffered from frigidity, while Kinsey found it to be 75 per cent. Hardenberg's figures have a very wide range from 10 to 75 per cent."

"An erotic zone always could be demonstrated on the anterior wall of the vagina along the course of the urethra."

"Analogous to the male urethra, the female urethra also seems to be surrounded by erectile tissues like the corpora cavernosa. In the course of sexual stimulation, the female urethra begins to enlarge and can be felt easily. It swells out greatly at the end of orgasm. The most stimulating part is located at the posterior urethra, where it arises from the neck of the bladder."

"If there is the opportunity to observe the orgasm of such women, one can see that large quantities of a clear transparent fluid are expelled not from the vulva, but out of the urethra in gushes. At first I thought that the bladder sphincter had become defective by the intensity of the orgasm. Involuntary expulsion of urine is reported in sex literature. In the cases observed by us, the fluid was examined and it had no urinary character. I am inclined to believe that "urine" reported to be expelled during female orgasm is not urine, but only secretions of the intraurethral glands correlated with the erotogenic zone along the urethra in the anterior vaginal wall. Moreover the profuse secretions coming out with the orgasm have no lubricating significance, otherwise they would be produced at the beginning of intercourse and not at the peak of orgasm."

"The erotogenic zone on the anterior wall of the vagina can be understood only from a comparison with the phylogenetic ancestry. In the most commonly adopted position, where "the lady does lay on her back," the penis does not reach the urethral part of the vaginal wall, unless the angle of the erected male organ is very steep or if the anterior vagina is directed towards the penis as by putting the legs of the female over the shoulders of her partner."

"The anterior wall of the vagina along the urethra is the seat of a distinct erotogenic zone."

Dr G was one smart dude. Thirty years later, Dr. Grafenberg's work was resurrected, the now famous spot he talked about in his article was christened the Grafenberg spot or G-spot for short.

The G-spot is located about 2-3 inches inside the vagina on the outside or anterior wall. That is it – no mystery, no nothing – that is the G-spot. It is not like the lost city of Atlantis or some beautiful, secret area run by the CIA. You can imagine your partner's G-spot as almost opposite her clitoris but below the surface on the inside anterior wall of her vagina. When you have felt your way around in the vagina, you'll get to know the G-spot, as "bump" surrounded by the smooth fleshy anterior wall. The "bump" will feel ribbed, almost like the roof of your mouth. Memorize the first sentence of this paragraph.

When you have some time, perform an Internet search for the keyword – G-spot – look through the search results. You find articles from respected professors, so called authority magazines and publications about *"The G-spot supposedly is a small, highly sensitive area on the anterior (front) wall of the vaginal."* Or you find questions from some poor guy asking about female ejaculation ...is it real? Is it dreaming? It's sad when some of these doctors are still standing around scratching their ass and wondering where the hell they went and hid that damn G-thang.

Can you imagine, a bunch of supposedly educated gorilla doctors sitting at a bar discussing the existence, or non-existence of the G-spot? All they have to do is find a willing partner, arouse her, stick a finger in her pussy – and there it is – about two to three inches in, on the anterior wall. Hmmm ….

Ladies, you should not feel too bad if your lover is a tad dumb when it comes to your bodies. Number one, there are no universal "owner" manuals taped to anyone's ass and number two it seems that some of the best sex researchers in the world wouldn't know your clit from your ass if it weren't for your titties being where they are!

Occasionally I get e-mails from couples that are not able to find the G-spot. The first piece of advice I give, is for the lady to get sufficiently aroused before her partner goes poking around looking for the G-spot. Whatever gets her going - watch a steamy x-rated movie, read a sexy story, talk dirty to her, tie her up, etc. Once her love juices are flowing – then it's show time.

An un-stimulated G-spot is only about the size of a

pea and feels kind of like a dry roasted peanut shell. As the G-spot gets aroused and stimulated it swells to the size of a small walnut, giving you the clue that you not only found the spot but that it likes you! When the spot has swelled, the lady is in the big O zone and with more erotic play; you will make her body sing.

In technical terms, the G-spot is a bundle of nerve clusters that trigger natural painkillers within a woman's body. These painkillers are the same endorphins that release during childbirth. The nerve endings are concentrated beneath the surface of the skin in a protective bundle, which allows for sensitivity and ability to handle fondling.

Ladies, I recommend you experiment and explore your body. Learn where your hot spots are before you let your lover explore. This way you can advise her (or him) where those spots are and what to do with them. Not finding the spot and not knowing what to do with it can lead to frustration and disappointment.

To find the G-spot, place one or two fingers inside your vagina while you are squatting. Put your finger in a fishing-hook position and rub. Some women find it useful to press against the lower abdomen in order to ensure better contact to the G-spot. When the G-spot is swollen, your outside hand can feel it pressed against your inside fingers.

You are able to stimulate your G-spot yourself; the problem with stimulating solo is that your arm and fingers run out of steam. You will be able to make yourself G-gasm several times, but eventually you will become a puddle, out of breath and exhausted. With a FWB, you do not have to worry. Your FWB can keep going long after you are unable to continue from complete fatigue.

Ladies, first as stressed earlier, get her sexually aroused – very important. Don't ever stint on foreplay. Yeah, I know that you want to jump right in and get your fingers wet. Take your time; get her going first before you go G-spot hunting.

To locate the G-spot, face your FWB while she is lying on her back and insert your index or long middle finger into her vagina. Then crook it upward toward yourself in a "come here" motion, sliding your fingertip along the top of the vagina until you find an area that is rougher than the rest of the vaginal wall. Make sure you have your fingernails clipped short before you do this - sharp fingernails will definitely spoil the moment. This rough or slightly ridged area is the G-spot, and touching it the first time, will often cause a woman to react with surprise and pleasure.

THE G-GASM METHOD

OK, does everybody know where the G-spot is?

One more time – everybody together: The G-spot is located about two to three inches inside the vagina on the outside or anterior wall.

Thank you! Very good - let's ride!

Now that we know where the G-spot is – it is time to have some fun. I have had great success with this Method; the most important thing you can remember is that every woman is different. No woman has the same attitude towards this type of play. Take it easy – relax, have fun and make it fun for your partner. Communication is key; encourage her to talk.

Surprisingly, many sex manuals do not teach or even talk about direct G-spot stimulation and G-spot orgasms. Everyone has heard about and knows about the G-spot; yet many researchers and so called experts, still refer to it as the "elusive" or "mythical" G-spot. Trust me, the G-spot is where I told you it is. Ladies, I know that some of you will want to guard this Method as a secret, so that you get all the hotties, but please; help spread the word. There are plenty of women out there that need satisfying. Soon, you will be able to satisfy any woman, any time and give her as many G-gasms she wants.

Despite both spots offering the ability to create mind blowing orgasms the G-Spot is very different from the clit. In the beginning, you might treat the two in a similar fashion with some soft touching and light rubbing. However, when you have stimulated the G-Spot enough to get it going, that is when the real fun begins. A good guideline to remember will be to show the clit some mercy but to be merciless when it comes to the G-Spot! Within reason, most women will appreciate a harsher approach to the G-Spot.

BACK TO NIKKI'S HOT HOLE...

You remember Nikki – she was my hot little FWB tied face down on my bed with her pussy dribbling wet.

Nikki's ass was still twitching up in the air. Nikki nodded meekly as I continued to play with her lips, spreading them apart and fingering her love hole.

I kept working my hand between her legs. She was dripping with excitement and her whole body was trembling. I slowly slid my thumb inside and I reached around until I found what felt like a soggy walnut.

"That's it ... that's the G-spot," I thought to myself.

I started to rub it back and forth with my thumb. Nikki was going insane. Her ass kept twisting and squirming back towards my hand.

Nikki let out a gasp and moaned, "Oh my God - that is unbelievable. A little to the right - ohhhh yeah. That's the spot."

She was gyrating and moving like I had never seen before. I kept at it, back and forth with my thumb, then in a circular motion, then back and forth again. Nikki was going crazy. Good thing her hands were tied or I would never have been able to hold her in place. She was on the verge of climax. Her pussy muscles were clenching and pushing back against my thumb with every move.

She was encouraging me as I moved my thumb with even more force. I really got into it. Her legs clamped tightly around my hand and she lifted her ass off the bed as she gave a loud, drawn out, moan. She was totally out of control, and in the throes of a G-gasm, a huge one, and she wanted my thumb to press harder against her sweet spot. I kept my attention on the prize, careful to keep up the stimulation so I could prolong her peak as long as possible. When she could take no more, she started to come hard, pushing back up against my hand. Her G-gasm was as intense as it was long.

"OhhGawdyesSSSSSS...YESSSSS...," Nikki moaned.

"That was unbelievable," mumbled Nikki.

I gave Nikki a minute or two to catch her breath then again started to rub her G-spot with my thumb. We continued on that way for about an hour. It was very erotic to watch her respond to my incessant G-spot rubbing. At one point, Nikki focused enough to turn her head and look at me. She had this look of excitement, panic, shock, fear, thrill and exhilaration all at once and not necessarily in that order. It was almost as if she did not know what was going on. Nikki had at least ten mind blowing G-gasms that night – not sure - I lost count. I could not tell you how many times I came just watching her and touching myself with my free hand when I could.

"Holy fuck - what the fuck? How did you do that?" Nikki asked, totally dazed but able to form a few words now.

I carefully untied her, kissing her wrists when the silk slipped away. She got up to go to the bathroom and her knees buckled. She gave me a strange look and managed to make it to the bathroom and then back to the bed.

After a short nap, she asked, "What did you use on me? And why did you wait until now to do what you just did?" Nikki asked.

"Well, maybe while you were on vacation I did some research on how to please a woman," I said half jokingly.

She did not believe that I had not used some sort of a battery-powered toy on her. But after she sifted through the sheets and under the bed, she realized it was all just my thumb and I.

"Whatever secret of the universe you found out about sex, you ought to write a book about it," she said. "And count me in for any hands on research."

NO SEX TOYS NEEDED

Nikki thought that I was using some kind of a battery-powered toy. She did not realize that my thumb did all the action. I kind of leaned back and made it appear that I did that to all my woman. In reality, that was the first time I had implemented the G-gasm Method that I had formulated from all the research I had done on the G-spot.

We spent the next few sex sessions perfecting her G-gasm experience. We wanted to see how many G-gasms she could stand without needing to stop and got to around 50-something in a five-hour sexual marathon. Since that time, I have seen some naturally multi-orgasmic women handle as many as 100 G-gasms quite well. It all depends on the woman. The farther along we went the more comfortable and knowledgeable about the process Nikki became.

"Why don't all gals know how to do what you just did," Nikki asked. "Well, all don't get a manual on how to please women at birth, ya know?" I said defensively.

"You ought to write that manual," Nikki said.

THE G-GASM METHOD

I am going to teach you how to please a woman. You will make her cum like never before. Kissing is nice, sucking their breasts is nice, nibbling on their clit is nice but you are going to learn how to give a woman G-gasm after G-gasm.

My partner(s) have blown their minds to a level that they never believed possible. The intensity, number and duration of both arousal and orgasms have increased exponentially compared to traditional and so-called "tantric" techniques.

While I have had great success with the Method, the most important thing you can remember is that every woman is different. If you move into dating and sexual types of relationships assuming that all women are the same, you are going to be mistaken. No woman has the same attitude and anatomy. While their anatomy may indeed be similar, they are not all the same, not by a long shot, and good communication is the cornerstone of great sex.

Later on, we will discuss variations of the basic G-gasm Method. Some of these variations will work better for you than others and will bring different results with various women. Some women will not have any huge orgasms but they may enjoy the intimacy and still receive enormous pleasure. Again, it just depends on the woman. Either way, plan to spend the first evening exploring her body.

Prepare your hands for this erotic experience. Scrub your hands well. Long manicured fingernails may look good, but not for what you are about to do. Keep the nails short and filed smooth. NO FAKE NAILS – many hospitals and doctors offices have banned the use of fake fingernails in the work area. Apparently, there is some doubt as to the cleanliness of the area beneath the fake nails. Why take a chance?

Long manicured fingernails may look good, but not for what you are about to do. Keep the nails short and filed smooth. Before you begin the activities, to help prevent rough, dry hands in any weather, be sure to routinely massage your favorite hand cream thoroughly into your hands. The massaging action stimulates blood circulation throughout the hands and promotes the absorption of conditioners into your skin. Apply your cream often, especially after washing your hands or after submerging them in water. FWBs will really appreciate your prep work.

For anal play, those that want a little "protection" there are a variety of products named "Finger Gloves," "Finger Cots," "Finger Caps" etc. that provide a thin layer of protection between your finger and Honey's butt hole. Do an Internet search for any of the above words and you will easily find them.

RULES

There are only two actual "rules" for the G-gasm Method.

Rule number one is to have the lady use the bathroom before you begin. Stimulation to the G-spot will give her the sensation that she needs to urinate. However, if she knows she just did, it is less likely to bother her. The urination sensation does not last for a long time, though you don't want to end up having a stream of her urine land on you. You water sports gals might not mind this; it would be a deal breaker for most!

Set the mood. Some candles and sexy music really set the tone. Barry White has some music to G-gasm by. Barry White's impossibly deep and sexy voice, one of the most recognizable in music and his satiny love songs will bring any woman to her knees. Although after a while, her screaming with joy will drown out any music.

Rule number two is probably more important than rule number one is. Start with foreplay – kissing, touching, a back rub – whatever the two of you are in the mood for. Do everything you normally would do to turn her on, do not go directly to the G-gasm Method. This is essential; you must get her going first. This is especially important the first few times you attempt G-gasms. Lots of oral, dip your tongue in her for a bit, try different positions, more oral, with nibbling and kisses and only then when she is about to burst, try the G-gasm Method. She should be fully stimulated and the whole vagina area engorged with her at the point of begging for more.

Some gals like to give their ladies an oral clitoral orgasm first, I recommend that you bring her close to orgasm, but don't let her cum. Use your talents and toys to bring her to the edge of orgasm over and over again. Many women are the one-orgasm types; their bodies trained and satisfied after one orgasm. Skip the clitoral orgasm; make her desperate for sexual release. If she is moaning, dripping wet, and almost incoherent she wants to cum so much, now is the time to go G-spot thwacking full-time.

Have her lay on her stomach with her rear up in the air and her face leaning against some pillows. Make sure to have her legs at a comfortable width apart. Put a couple of pillows under her hips to get her tush up in the air. Position yourself at her side or between her legs.

Insert your thumb, thumbprint side down, in her pussy. Press the thumb downwards so that you are pressing towards the pillows under her hips. You will find the G-Spot right about where your thumbprint is. I know it sounds simple, because it is! There really is nothing to finding the G-spot. Keep in mind everybody's body is different. If she looks, or says she is uncomfortable, back off for a while, go back to doing "comfortable" things. You can always try again later or the next session. The first time is the hardest – after that, it is easy to find and play with the G-spot – insert thumb, press down (this is with the lady on her stomach, butt up).

Feel around for a smallish, rough bump that is bigger than a pea. The size will depend on the woman and the amount of foreplay. As she becomes more and more excited and the G-spot is stimulated, it will grow in size to about the size of a small walnut. The G-spot is going to feel rougher than the smooth texture of the inner vagina walls.

Now that you found the spot, with your thumb, start rubbing. Start to rub in a back and forth or side to side motion. At this point, the key thing to remember is not to rub it too hard. You will be able to feel the spot thicken and grow against your thumb. Once this happens you will be able to increase your movement and get rougher with it. Rub it, as if you are trying to get a stain off your jeans.

Any gal that treats the clit rough will usually get a slap in the back of the head. After a clit stimulated orgasm, be it manually or with the tongue, even look at her clit and she will push you away. The G-spot is different. Once triggered and excited, do not treat it as a clit. In the excited state, the G-spot likes abuse – treat it rough. Be gentle with the clit – be rough with the G-spot.

As the G-Spot continues to swell, she will get the feeling that she has to urinate. However, that was the reason for having her take a pee beforehand. I always ignore the request. The feeling will go away in a little while.

When the G-Spot gets excited and swells, it puts pressure on the bladder giving the woman a sensation of needing to tinkle. This feeling only lasts for about 30 seconds, and then subsides. Many newbie women become uncomfortable at this point; I assure you the feeling will change to a highly sexual pleasurable feeling.

While many women don't have to be asked to talk, and are more than willing to tell you how to rub their G-spot, I have been with just as many who need that little extra push to talk. To find out if you are in the right spot, just ask. You may find she wants you to move to the left or right. She might want you to be rougher and faster or slower and softer. Try rubbing side to side, up and down, "punch" it, rub round and round, tap the spot like a tiny drum, poke at it like you are trying to push it, jab at it like you are trying to pick it up with a fork, press on it with no movement, bring out the dentist's drill, vacuum cleaner, or chainsaw ... whatever it takes.

After a few minutes you should hear the mind-blowing madness which will be your woman having a G-gasm. The first time I watched this I could not believe my eyes. My life changed with one G-Gasm! She'll be bucking and pushing against your hand with all she has, moaning and screaming, she'll cum so hard she may squirt all over your hand.

To be able to give a lover that much pleasure is the best feeling ever. After the initial bombshell, your lover continues on to even greater pleasure as you press on the G-gasm Method. That is why I wrote this book, to teach others how to discover and explore the G-spot - a guide - to delve into the world of G-gasms.

Not everyone will have quick, fast and successful results — some couples will have staggering G-gasms within minutes — other couples try everything short of sacrificing a goat — us girls are not the same. The couples having trouble need to be persistent, patient and eventually they will be like "WOW – WHAT THE FUCK – THAT WAS AMAZING." Once the first G-gasm is unleashed, all hell breaks loose. Whatever the immediate results are, remember that getting there is 90% of the fun.

A word of warning: Never try this Method with your lady sitting on your face. If you do not drown from the pussy juice, you will certainly have a broken nose.

CUNNILINGUS AND THE G-GASM METHOD

Her lips slid up and down my clit slowly. One long finger pushed in and out of my cunt in time with her mouth. I sighed and threaded my fingers in her hair. I did not need to guide her. She was so damn good at this - she was an older waitress and I was a newbie bartender.

Skyla was about 45, hard to tell, and that question is never asked. She had a few lines around her eyes and a few strands of gray peppered her shoulder length chestnut hair, but she was in great shape. I had dated girls who were probably half her age that didn't have as nice a body as Skyla did.

I had girlfriends who gave great oral, but not like this. Skyla would pause her sucking to lick and tease my swollen folds with the tip of her pink tongue. She would wink at me when she saw me smile, and then rim my opening before diving in. Skyla had the technique down pat.

She had a way of looking at me while I was mixing drinks – almost as if she wanted to rip my uniform shirt and vest off, throw me on the bar and abuse me.

I was working as a bartender in a place called "The Gold Rush." My boss hired me as a trainee bartender, working the day shift, and this was my first time on the night stint. At first, Skyla did not really strike me as being hot as much as her personality was cool. We worked together all night, her ordering drinks for her customers and me preparing them and placing the cocktails on her tray.

Whenever she approached the service bar area, she would say, "Ordering ... cocktails."

She would always emphasize "cock." I wondered if she had seen the slight bulge in my pants since I wore my strap-on cock to work. I had gotten used to wearing it and did not think anyone would notice that I was packing.

As I would get her order ready, Skyla would wait patiently with a cute little smile on her face. Skyla reminded me of my girlfriend's mother. She always said she had to hide her mom when I was around, which was true because her mom was hot. She was not safe.

We closed the bar around 2 AM that night, or I should say early that morning. We were all a little tired from the late night and I was going crazy trying to figure out if Skyla really was flirting with me. I lived close by, so I took the plunge and asked Skyla if she wanted to stop over for a beer and unwind a little before she headed home.

"Sure, I'd love to stop over for a cocktail," she said as she gave me a coy little smile. There it was again. My gaydar could not be far off, could it? If it was, all I had to lose was a little dignity. The prospect of possibly something more with Skyla was worth it.

When we got to my place, I cracked open a couple of beers and we sat down on the couch. It was amazing how easily we carried on a conversation about anything and everything. We spent a little while talking about that night's customers and then we just sat for a few minutes without saying anything.

I opened my mouth to ask Skyla if she wanted another drink and before I got a word out, she leaned over and kissed me. It was not a quick peck on the lips, but a slow, deep kiss that left me breathless and ended too soon.

"Whoa ... these older woman do not mess around," I quietly thought to myself.

I was not about to pass up the invitation. I reached over and started to unzip the back of her dress. She batted my hands away, saying that she could do it faster. She only had her black work dress on, and that was easy for her to take off. Her black bra was next and there she was, standing in front of me with only her panties on. I was still struggling with the buttons on my shirt; I was too busy looking at her. Her panties were black lace and so skimpy that the "how to wash" label was the biggest part on them. They were last to go tumbling to the floor.

"You can take off your clothes now and save time or wait for me to do it," Skyla laughed.

As she waited for me to get undressed, she played with her brownish-pink nipples. She rolled them gently in her fingertips, giving them a squeeze now and then and plumping them while I watched. My own nipples hardened in response. She slid one of her hands down her stomach to the vee between her legs. Her cute little bush, was trimmed to what I call a "landing strip," was shaved along the bikini line and both sides, with a neat, trim line of hair down the middle. It was awesome.

Her index and middle fingers traced her puffy pink lips. She pushed open her entrance and slid two fingers inside. I pushed and pulled off my clothes, not caring if I tore my bar uniform or not. I just wanted to be where those two fingers had just disappeared.

Skyla sat back down next to me on the couch. With her two fingers still in her pussy, she reached for my strap-on with her free hand. She grabbed the base of the dildo and worked it against my mound, knowing that would put the most pressure on my clit. My hips arched up off the cushion.

My clit was throbbing and I was getting wetter by the second. Skyla wiggled one finger under the leather straps and dipped out some of the moisture.

"Ohh," Skyla moaned delightedly and leaned forward to lick off her finger. "I love that."

Then she started to work on my cock. Her hand slid up and down unhurriedly, grinding the dildo against my center. Slowly, she raised her head and reached for my breast. Cupping the soft underside, she flicked the nipple with her tongue. I sighed, my senses on overload. My hands were restless though, and I could not stop them from wandering. I stroked her shoulders, her breasts and the soft skin of her inner thighs.

Skyla removed her fingers from her entrance so that I could get my hand between her legs. She looked up at me and leaned over to kiss me. I brought one arm around her soft shoulders and pulled her towards me. We fell back with Skyla on top of me, our lips locked together. I put my hands on the cheeks of her firm, well-rounded ass and pulled her up to straddle me. She started to grind her hips as I let my tongue part her outer lips, tasting her sweet, salty essence for the first time. I swirled my tongue around her folds before settling down to a steady pace.

"You know, it might not be such a bad idea if I try the G-gasm Method on her while she's on my face," I hungrily thought to myself.

Why did that thought cross my dirty little mind? Oh yeah … I know why. I was thinking I am going to be a butchly stud and hook Skyla on G-gasms. Hell no - everything started going south from that brilliant idea.

Funny thing was, while I was tongue fucking her and thinking about it, she begged me to put a finger in her. I did not hesitate; I was about to drive her crazy. With my tongue lashing away at her clit, I first stuck my index finger in her pussy, and then added my middle finger. It was the perfect position. All I had to do was the "come here" motion and there was the G-spot, the size of a small walnut, ready for rubbing.

I started touching Skyla with some light back and forth rubbing action, then switched to opposite strokes similar to walking on her G-spot. She loved it. The more I stroked, the more she started to move her hips. Skyla was humping my face hard, but I did not want to stop, knowing how much Skyla was enjoying herself. As I rubbed and licked her, I could feel the flood of moisture pouring from her. She was getting more and more excited and my goal of G-gasming her was about to happen.

I started getting a little concerned though when she was rocking on my face, oblivious that I was down there. "Hey wait a second, look down, there's a face down here," I was thinking. Before long, she was thrashing and screaming in G-gasm delight. When she finished and could breathe normally, she pulled me up then began to lick my lips and kiss me deeply. She broke off and whispered, "I love the way my pussy tastes on you."

When Skyla regained her senses, I eased her off me and tried to sit up. I felt a little dizzy, and it was not all from the sex. My nose was throbbing and a small trickle of blood began. Skyla looked like she was going to faint. That meant I could not, since one of us might need to drive me to the hospital. Besides, fainting would ruin my newfound status as a stud.

"I am sorry … so sorry … I do not know what came over me but I just could not control myself," Skyla apologized.

"That's okay," I told her, grabbing some tissue from the box on the coffee table and holding it beneath my nose.

Well sure enough, next day I went to the doctor and he had to reset my nose. I had to wear a splint for five days. That was attractive. I could tell my friends I got into a fight at the bar, but they probably would not believe me. The truth was even less believable. Nevertheless, I did learn one important lesson. Never do the G-gasm Method while a woman is sitting on your face.

THE NEXT LEVEL

After the first G-gasm, you can trigger additional G-Gasms within seconds to a minute. After she cums the first time, start rubbing again, just as hard as before. The G-gasms will happen repeatedly. Of course, each woman has a different tolerance for this, so you will want to watch it carefully. Some women cannot take the rigorous abuse of her body so often. If she cannot stand many G-gasms, don't worry, because as sessions continue, the need and ability to achieve multiple G-gasms seems to progress. You will have her experiencing 10, 20 or more G-gasms per session in no time. Again, do not be gentle – unless of course she asks.

When you have her at the exited point – the one where

she just experienced a G-gasm - DO NOT STOP. The whole idea of using the Method is that you can keep going. Wait until you see her reaction when you make her G-gasm for the first time, give her a few seconds rest, then keep going.

Now that she knows the feeling, it will be easier and easier to make her G-gasm repeatedly. The way to really blow her mind is make her G-gasm like that for 30 or 60 seconds straight, and then give her a rest to catch her breath and then start again ... and again ... and then some more.

It is like finding the key to the vault. Her body will know what it feels like from then on. Marathon sessions will be fun, but "quickies" in mall parking lots, or before breakfast are a scream too. Once the vault has been opened, reaction time can be almost instantaneous if she is horny and you have 30 seconds or so to get your thumb in there and give her a good rub.

Gals, this is much better than just FUN. Most women do not have any idea that they are capable of such sexual energy and multiple orgasms. After five or six G-gasms, they start to look at you with amazement. Like, "How the hell are you doing that to me?" I do not give them any mercy. I torture them with G-gasm after G-gasm.

FEMALE EJACULATION / SQUIRTING.

This lady is a freak of nature – "thar she blows ... " http://g-gasm.com/female-ejaculation.htm. From what I have seen, about half of women do **not** ejaculate. I emphasize that because many ladies fear they have failed, even though they just had 30 or more G-gasms, but didn't leave a bucket of cum on the bed sheets. There are women that do ejaculate and there are women that ejaculate sometimes and some that never squirt.

Like mirages, rainbows, shooting stars and other nature masterpieces, female ejaculation has provided amazement and controversy. Many woman and researchers believe that because the fluids expelled during female ejaculation come from the urethra, that really the woman is experiencing loss of bladder control. In other words – she peed a little.

Men take ejaculation for granted. It is the "runny-prize" of sex – and the source of their future heritage. The only conceivable purpose of female ejaculation is for pleasure – very intense pleasure at that. The G-gasm Method can produce ejaculation when performed on a willing partner.

In some porno movies, there is a scene where the woman is ejaculating a clear or milky fluid. Is it real pussy cum? Is it trick editing? Is it pee? That is a lot of questions … I think it is real.

I did a lot of research on female ejaculation, or squirting. I studied videos of women cumming, and I have read scientific articles, but nothing works better than hand-on research to figure out how to please a woman.

The tissue surrounding the female urethra fills with blood during sexual arousal, as the penis does in men. This results in the tissue becoming firm to the touch. Researchers believe that female cum is produced by the Skenes glands. Skenes glands are located in the urethra. These glands are similar in makeup to a man's prostate gland. Female cum is made of prostatic acid phosphatase, the same chemical secreted by the prostate gland and found in semen, minus the sperm of course. This indicates that a woman's ejaculation is similar in composition to semen.

Woman who experience G-gasms enter the wonderful world of "squirting." Not all women, all the time experience ejaculation, some experience it sometimes, some women never squirt. Most females have the ability to ejaculate, but often do not and usually squirting is a taboo subject and not discussed openly. When was the last time you heard of anyone discuss "depositing **her** load" over a few drinks?

In the past, medical doctors told ladies seeking advice about bodily fluids that they are incontinent, rather than told they are ejaculating. That led to shame and humiliation. What girl would want to be known as a bed wetter? Instead of enjoying the ejaculation sensation, many women believed they had "golden-showered" their partner. Many thought they had been "golden throated" while giving oral to their lady friend. Many females will admit to having had an experience where they believed they had "leaked" during sex. The feeling of ejaculating is similar to peeing, a shower of warm wet liquid and a feeling of release.

Gals, be prepared for the flow of ejaculate. If you are into "water sports," this is going to be a huge turn on for you. Do not react like "what the fuck is that -- did you piss yourself?" because that will make it embarrassing for both of you. It is a normal body function. Make your lady feel comfortable, or she will dry up like a mud puddle and so will your sex life. You laugh, but I swear, if she thinks she peed herself during sex, she will lose her sexual high completely.

Ladies, you will be amazed at the amount of fluid your body can produce. Up to two cups of expelled ejaculate can slather your sheets during a G-gasm session researchers say. The amount varies, as does the force of ejection. Sometimes, your hand will get soaking wet, and other times her spunk will bathe the soles of your feet. How awesome is that?

This is a new slant on the question of "who sleeps on the wet spot?" We are not talking about a small amount like a few teaspoons; we are talking about a couple cups of milkshake. The fluid can appear like watered down milk or can be clear.

SQUIRTING GUIDELINES

Most women can ejaculate but many do not. In the same way that all women can orgasm even though some do not ever achieve climax, be it through bodily or psychological blockage, or in-experience. Playing with her G-spot for hours at a time does NOT necessarily mean she is going to ejaculate. That happens with some ladies some times. Don't get bummed if it doesn't happen – she is still having G-gasms and having a good time. She doesn't need to squirt. Again, some women will squirt a little; some will gush a lot; some will not squirt at all; and some will shoot sometimes.

The ejaculation in woman is much more complex than men, but once they start they do not stop. Unlike men, there is more to follow. Give her a few minutes and she will be filling up like a Hummer's gas tank. Each subsequent G-gasm will produce a different volume of liquid in all directions and velocities. This can range from a trickle of one ounce to an almost a chaotic cupful. Don't worry about the juices drying up, there is always more.

Ejaculate fluid is different from the normal "pussy juice" or "love juices." Love juices are a natural lube for the vagina that appears with arousal. Squirting or female ejaculation comes from the urethra or pee hole.

Since female cum originates and emanates from the urethra, the fluid is mixed with a little pee. Men cannot pee and cum at the same time. When a man is about to ejaculate, the opening to the bladder closes, making peeing impossible. A woman on the other hand, (so to speak) is able to ejaculate and pee at the same time. Frequently that feeling of peeing and oncoming orgasm are confused. That is why I stressed earlier that your FWB should use the little ladies room, before you start your sexual activity. You do not want your lady to think about peeing – you want her thinking about G-gasms and ejaculations.

PC MUSCLES - KEGEL EXCERCISES

Kegel exercises are a good way to help control the peeing/ejaculating problem. Spend about a month training your muscles. This has the added benefit of greatly increasing the intensity of your orgasms, as the vaginal muscles become very strong with repeated Kegel exercises. These exercises strengthen a set of muscles known as the pubococcygeus or PC muscles. They are the muscles that both men and women use to stop the flow of urine. They are also the same muscles that contract and expand during orgasm.

Ladies, spend about 15 minutes a day for a month strengthening these muscles until they are so strong you can put your finger inside your pussy and grab it so tight you cannot physically remove it until you relax the muscles. You will have unbelievably strong orgasms.

A typical PC muscle workout: Start with tightening the muscles for 3 seconds, then relaxing. See how many times you can do this before they become tired. Next, start doing sets of five strong squeezes. Start with only a few sets, as with any exercise, you will work your way up to more sets. See Appendix A for more details on Kegels.

Once you work your way to three sets of 30 or more squeezes, your PC muscles are probably healthy enough for most purposes. The best part is that you can do these exercises anywhere. Do them while waiting in line at the grocery store; do them while at work, etc. Once you are skilled at Kegel exercises, you should be able to do them without anyone else knowing what you are doing.

SQUEEZE OUT FOR MAXIMUM FLOW

Getting your lady friend to squirt for the very first time is like obtaining a PhD in sexology. The building of the ejaculation feels like the desire to pee. As soon as the urethra starts to tingle, second nature kicks in and she contracts her PC muscles to stop the flow of urine. She must oppose the contraction and try to squeeze out, as if trying to pee. This is not an easy concept, in that contraction of the PC muscles will actually stop the ejaculation from building. As squeezing the base of the cock and thinking momentarily of Mickey Mantle's batting average postpones cumming in men, "squeezing in" postpones female ejaculation. "Squeezing out" instead of "squeezing in" is a major barrier for many ladies trying to ejaculate. Practice will overcome the barrier.

REMEMBER – SQUEEZE OUT

Be prepared, especially the first few times you use the Method, to see if she's a gusher or not. OK, you have been warned, don't forget to use the biggest towels you can find; you don't want your mattress to start smelling weird after a while.

VARIATIONS OF THE G-GASM METHOD

"MMMM... YYYEEAAHHH," Nikki moaned out, showing clear pride in herself for becoming so aroused from my thumb in her hole. "Jeez, this is so nasty, and I love it! I feel like such a slut," I heard Nikki whisper.

"You say that like it's a BAD thing," I laughed.

There are many different ways to use this Method. Having her bottom in the air – although that is a good thing – is not the only way to achieve G-gasms. The only thing that is going to limit you with this Method is your imagination. You have a new tool in your arsenal, use it and experiment with it.

You are introducing your lover to a fresh new horizon – you need to talk to her, because some things are about to change – you need to know your partner's wants and needs. I have been with women that loved G-gasms but emotionally just could not handle them on a frequent basis.

Keep an eye on your lady, especially the first few times you try the G-gasm Method. If your lover is used to being in control, then the total loss of control that comes with G-gasms may make her uneasy. She will still be able to enjoy herself, but women do lose control during these sessions. Some women get scared – scared at the intensity, frequency and total loss of control of the orgasms. Many FWBs will ask you to stop until they become comfortable with the Method.

This is where you have to decide whether it is time to hold her down and proceed or to go on to other activities. Often when she is at the "scared" point, her G-gasm is seconds away. If you can force a few more rubs, she will have no choice but to cum, and then you can repeat the process. Always be loving, understanding and supportive to your lady, but don't always let her call all the shots. Sometimes, even if you are usually a pussy-whipped girl-toy, this is a great time to slap her ass, pull her hair, tell her she's a slut and a whore and tell her to shut the fuck up and that you are in charge now. Pull this off and she will know the meaning of respect.

YOU ARE IN CONTROL

Lisa screamed and begged me to stop. She loved it and hated it at the same time. She loved it because it felt so good, but hated it because I was in total control. Unless you know there is real pain – give them one more when they tell you to stop.

Lisa, a petite blond with a cute little body and I were at a friend's party. We had only been hanging out for a very short time, and had not yet gone much farther than kissing. She was a fantastic kisser, but I had a feeling she was inexperienced with women otherwise. I was incredibly attracted to her and wanted to be the first to show her everything a woman's body had to offer.

All evening Lisa had been flirting more than usual, getting bolder with her teasing touches, soon I realized she was inviting me to take control. Not wanting to wait until we got back to her apartment, I grasped Lisa's hand and led her down to the basement to get away from everyone. She followed willingly and seemed to be glad for the chance to escape the crowd and loud music.

Have you ever had a G-gasm? I asked Lisa as we closed the stairway door, shutting out the rest of the world

"G-gasm?" she asked, waiting for my reaction to her lack of experience.

"G-gasms," I repeated casually. You know, a G-spot orgasm, I explained.

Lisa tried to keep a blank face, hoping that I would reveal more information without her having to ask. "I have never had an orgasm without my vibrator glued up against my clit," Lisa confessed.

I wrapped my arms around her waist and nuzzled her neck. I brushed soft kisses down to her shoulder and trailed my tongue back up to her earlobe, sucking it into my mouth and gently biting. Lisa shivered, and I felt my clit twitch in response.

"What do you think?" I asked with a teasing voice that made her smile. "You want to try. I promise you won't need a vibrator."

Without answering, Lisa pulled me closer to her and drew her lips close to mine. Her soft lips pressed hard against me, and my tongue parted her as I explored her silky mouth. I took that as a yes and slowly moved from her mouth down her neck.

Her hard nipples were straining against her t-shirt. I pinched them playfully, causing Lisa to let out a soft moan. Taking hold of the bottom hem, I peeled away her shirt that revealed perfect twin mounds covered by a lace bra. Lisa reached back, undid the snap and waited for me to reach out and hook my fingers in the straps. I slid her bra off her shoulders and let it fall to the floor, revealing beautiful pale breasts topped with deep red nipples.

I eased her down onto the carpet and straddled her waist. My hands slid from her stomach upwards to caress the underside of each breast, then cupped one in each palm. Her nipples grew even harder as I rubbed my hands in slow circles.

Lisa became either brave enough or excited enough to slip her hands under my shirt and do a little exploring of her own. I was not wearing a bra, a fact she soon discovered and her fingers brushed across my stiff nipples. As fantastic as that felt, I did not want to be distracted from giving Lisa her first G-gasm. Reaching up, I pulled her wrists from under my shirt and held them above her head as I slid a knee between her thighs.

I leaned down to kiss her and she bucked up against the pressure on her clit. She felt hot, excited, tingling against my thigh. I wondered if she liked having someone else take charge, and wanted that someone to be me.

My hands released her wrists and started making their way down to her waist. She moaned as I rose up and unbuttoned her jeans. With my tongue, I traced an imaginary path down her chin and neck, across her hard nipples, and around her belly button. I tugged her pants down her legs, tossing them behind us. Lisa's underwear followed next, her sweet, musky scent filling the cool room. She had goose bumps all over her body.

With my tongue, I resumed my earlier path and dipped into her navel before gliding down to the soft curls glistening with the evidence of her arousal.

"Oh, god," she whimpered, threading her fingers in my hair and pushing my head hard against her. Lisa moaned as I licked her folds and circled her clit.

I reached under her and grabbed her round cheeks, squeezing them and pulling her tighter against my face. She wrapped both legs around my shoulders and thrust her hips towards me. With the flat of my tongue, I lapped from her vagina to her clit, rimming both until Lisa whispered, "That feels so wonderful ... you are the best ever, you know that?"

"Yes, baby," I answered, "Now she's ready for some G-gasm action," I thought to myself.

I smiled, knowing how incredible this was going to be for Lisa. She was soaking wet and as I trailed my finger down her slit and back up again, Lisa let out a little whimper. I let my finger slide all the way inside her slick hole. I rotated it around in a circle and then pulled it out. Positioning myself where Lisa could see me, I slowly licked off my finger. I loved the way she tasted, a little bit salty yet sweet.

Deciding it was time; I reached in, found the G-spot and gave it the old come here motion. Lisa was ready; her G-spot was the size of a nice plump pea. Between my lips, Lisa's clit was swollen and pulsing, and her G-spot was plump and bloated on my fingertip.

With my finger, I rubbed her G-spot, trying out different degrees of pressure and adding some variety to my rubbing. Lisa, losing control as her hips arched up in the air. Finally, she exploded and her whole body seemed to strain against me. It was beautiful to watch. I gave her 30 seconds to regain her composure, and then started rubbing again.

Lisa looked up at me with this expression of pure panic and excitement. She was barely over her first G-gasm and already on her way to another. I continued rubbing. I felt her fingernails start to dig into my arms as she pushed her hips towards my inserted hand. I knew it was just moments before she would G-gasm again. I rubbed faster and furiously.

Her moaning and thrashing was getting increasingly louder which was a turn on for me. "I'm going to come again," she gasped. She started shaking as she threw her head back and screamed.

I gently withdrew my finger and replaced it with my tongue. Lisa was having a hard time catching her breath. Her face flushed a crimson red, her body covered in a thin sheen of moisture. I continued licking her until she started moving her hips in time with me. I reinserted my finger and found her G-spot, swollen to the size of a quarter. Perfect.

"I can't again so soon," Lisa whispered as she pulled away slightly.

"Yes you can Baby, one more time. I've got you," I encouraged her as I started rubbing her G-spot with one hand. I reached up and started rhythmically squeezing her nipple with the other hand. I wanted to push her past whatever limits she imagined she had and help her to feel safe giving up control and letting me show her how incredible multiple G-gasms are.

BDSM - YOU ARE SO NAUGHTY

If you want to crank things up a notch or two, add in a little BDSM activities during your G-Spot marathon. A few well-placed spankings with your hand or a paddle will do. In addition to this, tie her down and control how many G-gasms she has. What a nice little mixture; the kinkiness of a G-spot rubbing together with a little bit of submissiveness. However, always be careful and sensitive to the needs of your lover, because this might be too intense for some women.

"Don't you dare try and wriggle away from me," I warned Jasmine. With a hard smack to her bottom, I made my point. Jasmine moaned softly and I delivered another smack. Her cunt got wetter with every whack and my thumb slid up and down easily. Jasmine really craved some light spankings when we had sex. She loved it, and wiggled her ass to encourage more. I spanked her harder; I watched as her cheeks at first flushed, then turn blood red.

Up until a few months earlier, I had no idea about how hot spankings could really be. I had experimented with a slap or two on some particularly luscious asses before, but nothing to the extent that I shared with Jasmine. Jasmine changed all of my preconceived ideas about spanking. Jasmine was not her real name, to tell you the truth; I do not even remember her real name. It does not really matter though, because I will never forget her.

Jasmine was a thin Mexican beauty with dark brown hair. Besides the hair on her head and her eyebrows, she did not have a strand of hair on the rest her body, right down to her lovable little pussy. One day, Jasmine and I were in a bar having a drink and chatting. Out of the blue, she asked me what I thought about spanking during sex. The more she talked about it, the more excited she looked and that was enough to get me interested.

"The other day I was at a spanking blog, and as I read a few posts, my pussy got so fucking wet," she confessed to me. "Normally I would just masturbate, but something inside my head snapped. I thought to myself that it is time to stop reading and imagining, it was time to turn some of my fantasies into reality," Jasmine confided.

Right then a dozen mental images popped into my head, and I started to get wet myself. I was not very shocked that Jasmine was suggesting that I tie her up and spank her. I knew she was kinky and liked some of the rough stuff on occasion. Now, I am a nice butch. I do not go around beating the crap out of people, unless of course they deserve it. So as interested as I was in the thought of adding this new facet to our relationship, I told her I was a little afraid of hurting her.

Jasmine convinced me that this was something that she really wanted. After some more discussion, we agreed to try it. I had never been a complete top, but domination intrigued me.

We finished our drinks and headed back to my apartment. It felt a little strange at first. I was not certain if I was supposed to take charge immediately or what. To give myself time to think, I began searching for something to use as tie-downs. I found a silk tie I wore once on New Year's and decided that would do. Jasmine had followed me into the bedroom and was watching with amusement, her dark eyes sparkling. Realizing I needed to take control right then or it would never work, I walked up to Jasmine and stopped in front of her.

"How hard do you want me to spank you?" I asked Jasmine.

"I don't really know," she admitted. " I have never done this. I guess hit me hard enough to really experience the sensation of my ass being on fire," Jasmine replied.

"How many spankings should I give you?" I wanted to be clear on what she wanted.

"Let's just see what happens. Keep going until either I can't handle any more or your hand gets tired," Jasmine teased. I could tell she was a little nervous now that we were actually going to do this.

"Okay, that sounds like a plan," I agreed. "But we need a safe word for you. How about 'uncle'?"

"What is a safe word?" Jasmine asked, looking puzzled.

"A word you say that immediately stops all action," I explained. "Just in case you are screaming "stop, stop," but really mean "more, more." When you say "uncle" that is it; no more for real," I explained.

Jasmine agreed that this sounded like a good plan. "Start light and work your way up," Jasmine told me, winking, as she started to undress.

"No problem," I told her, winking back.

The real problem was thinking of where to tie her down. My bed was just a mattress, no backboard, so that would not work. Looking around the room, I spotted the roll top desk. Perfect. I could lean her across it and tie her wrists to the wood finials at the top.

"Put your wrists together," I demanded.

Jasmine complied and I wrapped the tie around her wrists and told her to stand in front of the desk. I grabbed a pillow from the bed to soften the surface for her and then pushed her forward. Raising her arms up, I secured the silk ends around the wood, pulling out the slack but not making it too tight.

Jasmine was able to move her legs, but her hands and arms were completely restrained. She closed her eyes. I could tell she was very nervous, yet also very sexually aroused. I wanted to see if the pleasure and pain thing was for real. I gently rubbed her smooth ass a few times until I could not take the anticipation anymore.

I lightly tapped her bare bottom with the palm of my hand. With each whack, my stroke grew stronger. Jasmine's hips were starting to rock back and forth. She seemed to be really enjoying it and that was a complete turn on for me.

"Wow this is incredible," I thought to myself. After a couple of hard strokes, I ran my thumb the length of her slit. She let out a low groan. Her pussy was drenched, the folds slick and hot. It was amazing to me. Aside from spanking, I had not even touched her yet. Normally I would have spent half an hour's worth of attention on her breasts and clit before she got this excited.

"This is making you wet, isn't it?" Jasmine nodded, her breathing ragged. I gazed at her body as I continued to stroke her. Her skin was flushed a light pink and there was a thin sheen of perspiration visible.

I inserted my thumb into her hot pussy, started to rub her engorged G-spot with one hand and continued to spank her with the other.

When I delivered a particularly forceful smack, Jasmine let out a startled scream. Finally, it was too much for her, and she yelled, "STOP!"

I paused for a second, giving her the chance to remember the safe word. When she did not say any more, I continued the rubbing and smacking. Jasmine was rocking back furiously. A few more slaps landed on her now brick red ass and she was trembling. She began to beg me to let her come.

"Rub harder... please. I need to come." she managed to cry out.

I whispered, "Are you sure you're ready to come baby? Because I'm in charge here and I'm not convinced yet."

I let out a silent chuckle at her groan of frustration. I could feel the evidence of her arousal coating my hand and I bent down to taste it. This surprised Jasmine, and she reeled back at the new sensation.

After only a few minutes, I was the one who could not take it anymore. I unzipped my pants and pulled out the strap-on cock I wore. It was Jasmine's favorite, bright blue and not too big. With one quick thrust, I buried the dildo to the base of the harness. We both moaned at the same time.

I slowly pumped in and out, knowing how good this was feeling to her as the dildo massaged her warm, slippery inner walls, especially the G-spot. It felt incredible to me, too. Every stroke put pressure on my stiff clit and I loved it. I worked in and out, enjoying the rhythm, but Jasmine needed more.

"Come on baby. Fuck me like you mean it," Jasmine challenged me, knowing how I would respond.

It was not long before my downward thrusts hitting the G-spot harder and faster brought Jasmine to a mind blowing G-gasm. Her legs shook and her wrists strained at the silk ties. But in only a few seconds, she wanted more.

"Come on baby. Fuck me harder," she dared me, even though she really was not in a position to be giving orders.

"You like this baby girl." I questioned her as I worked my cock deeper inside her.

"Yes. I like it! I like it! Keep fucking me - harder - harder! " She panted, rocking back and forth against me.

I teased her a little bit, slowing down, pulling out, then pushing in hard again. I gave her a few swift slaps on her ass making sure I had her complete attention. My clit was throbbing to the point of being painful and I knew Jasmine had to be close again too. I felt the first shockwaves start between my legs and shouted out.

"I am gonna come," I ground out as I arched against Jasmine.

"Do it, baby, come with me."

Jasmine was already falling over the edge again. Her pussy was clenching down on my strap-on, gripping it so tightly I could not move. She threw her head back and we both exploded together. I collapsed against her back, needing a few minutes to catch my breath.

When I felt her body relax a little, I slowly pulled out. Wrapping on arm around her waist to support her, I reached up and untied her wrists. Holding her in both of my arms, I let her heart rate return to normal.

"You're beautiful when you come baby," I whispered, almost as exhausted as she was.

"Uncle," Jasmine said softly.

WHAT IS EDGING

When you make love with someone, there are always going to be some happy accidents. Your partner carried away with excitement, bites a little too hard, but at just the right moment it feels incredible to. Or you just suddenly become inspired to try something you never considered doing before. That's how I discovered edging.

During spring break in my last year of college, most of my friends had flown to all the usual destinations. Jasmine went to Cancun, Nikki was at Daytona and Lisa was in New Orleans. I had always done Florida for spring break, which had become a little mundane. This year I wanted to do something else. It was my final chance to get a little wild before graduating.

As if on cue, a former girlfriend of mine named Jena got back in touch with me via telephone. She and I had dated over a year ago and it was one of the most incredible relationships I had had up to that point. I really thought I was in love, but convinced myself I was over her now. The last time we had been together she made it perfectly clear that it was about the sex, nothing else, and the sex was good enough that I readily agreed.

Jena called me at around eleven o'clock on a Friday night. She seemed to want to pick up right where we left off and was launching a full-on flirt with me over the phone. Pretty soon it turned into truth or dare, without the truth part, and eventually phone sex. I couldn't tell for sure just what was going on at the other end of the line, but from the sexy moans and sighs, she sounded like she was having fun.

The next day she called me again and invited me to visit her in Los Angeles. "Jena, if I come out to see you, it's only as a friend," I teased her. "You haven't lost your touch, even from a distance. However, don't have any false expectations. I am not sleeping with you."

"Yeah, yeah, I know. Last night was kind of a spur of the moment thing, for old time's sake. But it was fun, wasn't it? And it's not like I'm going to handcuff you to the bed once you get here." Jena replied.

"Huh?" I questioned, not sure, I had heard Jena correctly, although I hoped so. "What was that last thing you said?"

"Nothing," she answered, laughing. "Well sweetie, in a week you'll be skiing on the water instead of on snow wearing a parka."

"I'm not your Sweetie!" I reminded her.

"Yes dear, just a figure of speech," she said.

"Now, no hitting on me or getting me drunk and vulnerable. Definitely no kissing me the way you used to and wearing me down," I shot back knowing that is probably what Jena had in mind. She knew exactly how to make me crazy, and that is exactly what I wanted. We would talk a little, see the sights and get wet, just not necessarily in that order.

"I'll see you Tuesday at the airport in LA." Jena blew me a kiss over the phone before she hung up.

I got to LA Tuesday night. Jena picked me up at the airport, and after a quick tour of the city, we stopped at a local gay bar and she pulled me onto the dance floor. This was something new. I could not remember ever dancing with her when we dated. After she pressed her body against mine, sliding a thigh between my legs, I realized what I had been missing.

She moved against me in time with the music for three songs and I swear my heart and clit were pounding louder than the bass guitar. Suddenly she stepped back and smiled. Taking my hand, she led me to the car without a word and drove back to her house. It was around midnight, quiet except for the soft rustle of fabric as Jena started to unbutton her blouse.

"How about we take a shower together," Jena asked. "I'm a little overheated from that workout on the dance floor."

"Uh . . . well . . . uh . . . yeah, I would love to," I replied, caught a little off guard. I was used to Jena telling or showing me what she liked in bed, but she was never this open about it. It was a definite turn on for me.

Jena led me to the shower and adjusted the stream from the showerhead before slowly removing her blouse, then letting her skirt pool at her feet. My hands automatically reached for her breasts that were spilling out from a lacy peach colored bra, but she stopped me and finished undressing herself. Next, she took her time removing my clothes, pausing to brush over a nipple or rub my stomach, but never long enough to satisfy.

Stepping into the shower, she opened her arms and invited me to join her. I held on to her neck and looked at her in a new way as we let the warm water cascade down our exposed bodies. Soaping up a washcloth, gently she began to explore my body, pausing to trace the curve of a breast or the dip of my navel.

She softly ran her soapy hands down my back, running her nails along my spine. I pulled myself closer to her, feeling her hard, erect nipples rub against my own. I gave her a tender and sweet kiss. She moved one hand from my back down to my ass and the other hand to my left breast, squeezing them both firmly. Our kisses became hotter and more passionate as her fingers released my swollen nipple and trailed down my stomach, cupping my center. In unison, Jena pushed a soapy finger into my ass as she easily slid two fingers into my cunt. I began to shake uncontrollably as she stroked in and out. As incredible as it felt, I was not ready to come yet.

"Let me get your back," I managed to whisper. Turning her around, I took some soap from one of the wall-mounted canisters and lathered up. It gave me a moment to slow down and catch my breath. As I started rubbing her back, Jena closed her eyes, tilted her head back and told me how good it felt.

I pulled her towards me, as I reached around and cupped her breasts with both hands. Her breasts were the perfect size in my opinion. They filled my hands and I kneaded them gently for several long minutes. Working my way back around her waist, I grasped both cheeks of her firm ass and alternated between squeezing them together and pulling them apart slightly. Jena kept her eyes shut, her arms up in the air, and moaned in a sensuous, relaxed tone.

"That feels so nice," Jena said with my hands gliding over her hot, slippery skin. Her whole body was glistening, and not just from the shower.

Jena turned sideways to rinse off the soap but my hands continued to stroke her, one caressing her shoulders and neck with the other moved down over her stomach and hips, the feelings tantalizing yet gentle. I slipped my still soapy hand into the crack of her ass and my other hand between her legs. Threading my fingers through the curls, I explored her folds and was amazed at how ready she felt. Jena spread her legs just a bit to give me better access and I worked my hand harder.

I slipped one finger into her with my thumb pressed against her stiff clit. She shivered unexpectedly and arched her back slightly to get a better position. Jena encouraged me by grasping my wrist and moving along with me. "Mmmmm," she turned her lips towards me and whispered. "This feels great."

It was one of the most erotic things I had felt, working my finger inside her while she held onto my wrist. She was not guiding me or pushing, just hanging on for the ride.

Standing at her side, my fingers had a perfect angle to reach her G-spot. Jena's G-spot was the size of a quarter so I knew she was ready. Pulling out completely, I returned with two fingers. Jena sucked in a breath at the sensation but quickly started rocking against the added pressure.

Keeping my fingers stiff, I plunged in and out setting a steady rhythm that had her hips moving. My thumb gently caressed her engorged clit, but did not give her enough stimulation to come yet. I wanted to probe other places first.

My other hand was busy rubbing and massaging her ass. I worked a finger into the space between the cheeks and stroked up and down, stopping to rub small circles around the pink pucker there. On an upward stroke, I gently inserted the tip of my finger into that unexplored territory. Jena groaned as my finger slid in up to the first joint. She pushed back on it, automatically wanting to feel her ass stretch around it.

"Oh fuck, so damn tight," Jena moaned, stilling her movements as slick hidden muscles deliciously squeezed my finger.

I gradually worked my finger deeper into her tight hole, and she shivered as a wave of bliss flooded her body. She bit her lip as I finger fucked her ass. I reached to find her G-spot with my other hand. I started to stroke the now swollen spot in earnest, moving faster and harder. She cried out with my fingers rubbing back and forth over her G-spot, my thumb massaging her clit, and around the other side of her body, a finger working her ass.

I could hear the slick, wet sound of my fingers gliding in and out of her pussy. It all felt so good yet a little bit dirty.

"Is this what you want, baby?" I whispered the question into Jena's ear, which was close enough to my lips to suck the lobe in and nip gently. "Does this feel good? Do you like having my fingers in both your tight little holes?"

Jena did not speak, she only nodded while her hips were pumping and gyrating in time to my thrusts.

"You like having me fuck you this way, don't you? You have missed having me touch you this way. Say it, Baby, say it or I'll stop right now." It was an empty threat on my part, but Jena always used to love it when I talked dirty to her.

"Oh hell yes!" she spit the words out from between her clenched teeth. "Yes I like it! Yes, I have missed you, so fuck me any way you want! Oh my gosh … I am gonna …"

I stopped rubbing her G-spot as she approached climax. I pulled my fingers from her pussy and brought them to my face. I inhaled deeply, savoring the musky scent before tasting it. Jena opened her mouth and sucked one of my fingers between her lips, licking the juices off with her tongue. Watching her mouth move, it was almost as though I could feel her tongue swirling around my clit instead of my finger and I was going to come any second myself if I didn't get back to pleasuring her body.

Withdrawing my finger from her mouth, I reached back down to between her thighs and slid in easily. Jena spread her legs wider and thrust her hips towards my fingers picking up the pace we had moments ago. I started punching away at her G-spot and she immediately gripped my wrist again and urged me to move faster and harder.

My other hand's finger was still diving deep in her ass. Changing speed, I began to rub her G-spot a little rougher than before. A muffled moan burst from her when my thumb stroked her swollen clit. Spreading her legs, she moved in rhythm with me as I drew slow and sensuous circles around her flesh.

I leaned in and kissed her once, twice, three times before sliding my tongue between her soft lips. She groaned with delight and responded by gently sucking. I kissed my way across her jaw line and down her neck, taking the tender skin between my teeth and pulling. Jena released my wrist and reached for her rock hard nipples, pulling and pinching them.

Her G-spot, swelled to the size of a bottle cap as I rubbed it furiously. I could feel her squeeze my fingers with her pussy and ass, the inner muscles clenching in spasms.

"Oh, fuck, baby that it - Oh, shit that's it - Don't stop ... I'm done, I'm gonna come..."

Again, I pulled my fingers out of her pussy; I wanted to prolong the first G-gasm as long as possible. It was incredible being with Jena this way after over a year's time. Maybe we had both matured a little or maybe we just knew our bodies better. But this was the best sex we had ever had and I was not ready for it to end yet. I wanted to tease her a little longer, by bringing her right up to the edge of G-gasm, and then stop rubbing for a few moments. I knew that by doing this, the orgasms that followed would be almost intolerably intense and recur quickly - something to remember me by, at least.

Jena kept riding my finger in her ass. She rode slowly up and down, doing her best to draw more of my finger in her.

"Oh, god, that's good..." Jena let out, "More, keep doing it ... yes, give it to me …"

"You like having me fuck your ass, don't you?" I kept up the game of talking dirty. "But I want it all, baby," I told her as I thrust my fingers back into her pussy.

My fingers found her G-spot again and I started rubbing. I was ready to let her explode. Her pussy started to shake and convulse. Her breathing came in shallow pants, as she started moving in rhythm with my fingers. Waves of pleasure crashed through her body, each one stronger than the last. Her slick walls squeezed my finger as it moved within her. I quickened the pace of me finger fucking her ass with one hand and rubbing her swollen G-spot with the other. It was almost more than Jena could take, but I did not believe she really wanted me to stop.

She exploded into the wildest craziest G-gasm I had ever witnessed. It seemed to last forever. This G-gasm lasted for what seemed like several minutes. My fingers did not stop moving until Jena's cries faded and the jerky movements of her body stilled. Wrapping my arms around her, I pulled her close, holding her tight. Her body convulsed so intensely I could not help but ask her if she was all right.

When done, she whispered, "Yeah, I'm OK - Ooooh my GOD ... that was fucking unbelievable ..."

It felt great to be able to give Jena that much pleasure in a completely new way. It was like the first time we ever had sex, only much, much better. I had never known Jena to be multi-orgasmic, but she definitely was. Sometimes all it takes for a woman is discovering the G-gasm method. It is amazing.

Jena and I finished washing each other, dried off and headed for the bedroom. I never did get to see much of L.A. that weekend, but who cares?

WORKING THE G-GASM METHOD

♥ Peeing - the subject of most emails. Make sure she goes for a good pee before you start your activities, so she knows her bladder is empty. She will get that "I have to pee" feeling as the G-spot swells with excitement. That "I have to pee" sensation precedes huge multiple G-gasms and puddles of cum. Help her relax and accept the new sensations, mix it up with a little oral, while you are "training" the G-spot. Often the first G-gasm will happen when she least expects it. After that, it is easy to "rinse and repeat."

♥ After the first G-gasm, give her a short 10 – 30 second break, this gives her time to catch her breath but not long enough for her to come down from her high. Then proceed with more rubbing – the same way you did for the first G-gasm. Keep doing what you were doing – don't piss her off – she'll poke a hot stick in your eye when you are sleeping. If she is seriously overwhelmed and does not want anymore, this gives her the time to let you know.

♥ You are in control of her orgasms; you can allow them to come full on, or hold them back. Once you make her cum once or twice, you can continue this cycle until she begs you to stop, or until she goes into an orgasmic coma of sorts.

♥ If the woman you are with has an active job, you might want to save this activity for special events and weekends. I can guarantee that she will be sore and have a somewhat hard time walking when the next day rolls around.

♥ If there is not an immediate response from the lady, take it slowly; work her with foreplay so that she is as horny as you can make her. Work her orally or whatever gets her juices flowing and then try the Method again. If she still does not respond, go back to something else; get her near orgasm, then return to the G-gasm Method. You are in no rush – have fun.

♥ When rubbing, vary the pressure. Of course don't hurt your FWB, but it takes a firm hand and fingers, and a surprising amount of pressure to produce a G-gasm.

♥ This will become addictive to her. It will make your woman feel fulfilled and confident.

♥ Many women have expressed to me that a G-gasm is a mind-blowing experience. Their entire body receives a sense of relief. If a woman has never experienced this, you may want to give her more than a minute between each G-Gasm. Wait until she seems to have caught her breath. Once she can breathe normally again, it is time for round two, three, four, or ten.

♥ Do not worry about the size of your fingers; it is going to have little to do with the amount of pleasure she ends up receiving. Length and width has nothing to do with this. Instead, you will be concentrating on the amount of pressure you are using and not how much you are shoving inside her.

♥ Experiment with just slightly different positions of your finger(s). The G-spot is easy to miss, and if you are off just a bit the rubbing will still feel good for the lady, but won't produce G-gasms.

♥ Try edging, to increase the intensity just a little bit more; learn the flow of her G-gasms and stop before she has one. Start rubbing her and get her close to G-gasm, then stop. Give her a minute for a breather and then go back to rubbing. Leave your fingers/thumb inside her but do not move them. When you do finally rub her off, she'll buck her hips and grind back on your hand.

♥ If you have never experienced female ejaculation, it may appear that she is squirting something. Don't worry! It is not pee or anything. It is a good thing, especially for her! Some women become embarrassed after ejaculating the first time – they think they peed in bed – but it is not pee. With G-gasms, some ladies will ejaculate – go with the flow, so to speak. Bring a towel … or a bucket. Remember, keep rubbing past the "I got to pee" feeling, she is ready to G-gasm! We'll talk more about gushing later.

♥ Ladies, I know that you are going to try to do this Method on yourself. Many women have a hard time being able to create the proper level of necessary pressure to bring on the type of orgasms they could with someone else doing the rubbing. In order for you to hit your own G-Spot, you would need to slide your fingers inside yourself, and push them upwards and out; an awkward angle – maybe you could do it while squatting. There are some good toys on the market. Do a web search for G-spot vibrators at: http://G-gasm.com/toys

♥ Water based lubes sometimes help. Do a search at http://G-gasm.com/toys

♥ Once your lady has "graduated" a few G-gasm sessions, her body seems to know what to expect and not as much foreplay is required to trigger a series of G-gasms. You can warm her up a little, insert thumb/finger rub and give her three or 4 massive G-gasms. It is a great way for a little quickie before she heads off to work. She'll be smiling and glowing all day long.

♥ Most women are capable of G-gasms. Barring surgery and birth defects, all women have the correct "plumbing" in place to make G-gasms happen. This doesn't mean that the Method will work on all women 100% of the time. A combination of factors prevents G-gasms from happening. Fear, being the biggest culprit. Fear of "being dirty," fear of letting loose, fear of urinating and fear of losing control – these fears can be overcome. But birth defects, a cesarean section, hysterectomy or other surgeries may make it impossible to achieve G-gasms.

♥ Sex is not about the destination but rather the journey. If she's enjoying it, keep it up. With time, you will make progress. I receive countless emails from couples saying, "doesn't work …," "we can't …," "it seems that

...," or "didn't work." Later, all of a sudden I receive, "WOW ... unbelievable." Do not get frustrated and give up ... keep at it you will not be disappointed.

♥ Ladies, spread the word on the G-gasm Method. Think about it, what would happen if you, who experienced the ecstasy of G-gasms with a knowledgeable partner, had to move on to a new partner who lacked the necessary skills to help you achieve G-gasms? The same old, same old would not be good enough. You would have to teach her the skills; you would pass on the knowledge to your new lover. Some gals will take offense, but sex and what you prefer is part of everyday life that you share with your partner. Hell, you might even schedule some remedial classes if she was a slow learner.

MULTIPLE VAGINAL ORGASMS

The best part about this Method is that after the first G-gasm, the carry-over effect is real and may last for hours. Most women can achieve another G-gasm with only a few well-placed rubs. Wait 10 seconds to 30 seconds, rub a little more and it would all happen again ... and again ... and again. That is what makes this Method so awesome.

GALS, TRY THIS ... STRAP-ON SEX

After a few manual – meaning finger or thumb – G-gasms, position yourself between her knees, while she is on her back. Spread her knees apart and hold her still. Make sure she is wet, or lubed up, and insert the head of you strap-on in her pussy. Instead of thrusting like an exotic dancer, rock back and forth gently, aiming your dildo to stroke the top of her pussy. A dildo with an upward curve works best, so it rubs right up along the top, or front of the vagina, makes the sensation for her even better. You might want to push her knees up and back towards her to get a better angle.

After a few minutes of this, she will slip into another

world – maybe another universe. After her first G-gasm, she might appear to go limp - just kept going of course! Within perhaps 30 seconds, she will go into some scene from Psycho; she will buck uncontrollably. Hold onto her legs, you don't want her getting away, because you want to do it again, and again ... and then once more.

STRAPON WITH JENA

Jena and I stood next to the bed, quickly dropping our towels and becoming a heap of flesh, kissing and fondling each other passionately.

Fumbling around in my dresser draw, I found my strap-on and fastened it around my waist.

I bent one of her pillows in half and stuck it under my ass to lift my cheeks from the surface of the bed. What this does is it lifts your hips up and puts your dildo at an angle to where the lady can hit her G-spot. In order for her to do this, she has to lean towards you and then go at it. This allows the dildo to keep passing over the frontal wall of the vagina, where the G-spot is located.

Jena got on top of me and positioned herself over my strpon. She rocked her hot, wet pussy against my member. She closed her eyes as she lowered herself down on top of me. She braced her hands on my chest, and did sort of an "ocean wave" with her ass moving it in small circles. Soon after she started riding me, she let out a yelp as her pussy quivered around my dildo.

I was hitting her G-spot, because every in-stroke caused another squeal of delight. She arched her back and screamed to the ceiling, "Your cock ... it's making me cum ... I'M CUMMING ... I'M CUMMING ..."

Jena had about four or five G-gasms in the top position. I guided her off me and positioned her on all fours, with me behind her.

"Do you want this big cock in your wet juicy cunt? You like that?"

Once the G-spot is "alive," try the doggy-style position. On a psychological level, I think doggie style makes a woman feel dominated and over-powered almost a bit slutty, if that makes any sense. It is a "Butch" position, very dominating and animalistic, you know what I mean? Most girls love it when pumped from this angle; it is the best way to hit the G-spot with your tool.

Ask your FWB to prop some pillows under her hips, face down. Stand or kneel higher than her ass, and thrust downward and along the front wall of her pussy. "I love it when you hit me from behind," Jena said, as she positioned herself on her knees and elbows, arching her back to lift her ass high for me. I loved her ass, which she thought was excessively big, but she loved the fact that I enjoyed grinding against it.

My thick dildo plunged in and out of her; her pussy stretched out and clenched on to my tool. From this angle, each time I pushed into her, my thick head rubbed against her G-spot. Jena was completely under my control … and loving it. The thrusts became rapid, delivering almost a continuous orgasm, leaving Jena little recovery time. With one extremely hard push, Jena felt her entire body erupt in the most all consuming orgasm she had ever experienced in her life. Every cell in her body felt awesome. I owned every part of her at that moment.

G-GASMS FEEL LIKE ...

My girls have described them as:

"It felt like I had not come in three years, and was finally letting the entire year's worth of tension flood out of me at once."

"I completely lost all control of my body."

"A huge gush flowed out of my pussy – like in a porno film."

"Heavenly ... went on and on and on ... one long, continuous full-body orgasm. <Big sigh> ... I miss it already."

"One G-gasm, then another, another ... one after the other. I was amazed. I actually got terrified because I was out of control. I mean ... these orgasms were so different and intense from anything I had ever experienced. It wasn't local – meaning just in the vagina area – the G-gasms washed over my whole body."

"I have no idea how many G-gasms I had. When the G-gasms are happening, I could not tell you my name – never mind trying to count. Explosive, intense, very wet, throbbing, blurred thoughts, taut muscles, murmuring, shaking, white lightening, twitching for hours – those are some words to describe G-gasms."

"G-gasms are not ordinary orgasms – more like body orgasms that last, roll into one another and move me to another planet. Steady vigorous stimulation is the key and DON'T STOP (especially when I tell you to stop)!"

"I have never squirted like that before - wow wow wow.... very different kind of release."

"G-gasms are awesome … I worship your thumbs … I am addicted to G-gasms … I better insure your thumbs."

"Still walking funny." <Jasmine said this … she's a riot. >

EMAIL ...
WE GET EMAIL

I love e-mail. Please send me feedback on the contact form at: http://g-gasm.com/contact.htm I am constantly learning new tricks and am more than willing to help the couple that is having trouble achieving G-gasms.

The web site also has a discussion blog for anything G-gasm related. Please visit and post your questions and comments. Help spread the word. Millions of ladies need G-gasms. The G-gasms are coming ... the G-gasms are coming!

"WOW, THIS IS BETTER THAN FUN!"

"I am a middle-aged woman in a relationship with a lady around my age. We have been together for a few years. While she is willing and able to accommodate me sexually, she usually does not reach climax.

I felt like I tried everything to make her orgasm, then I learned about the G-gasm Method. I approached her about it and let her read your book. She was skeptical, but said we should try it. I had never tried this before so I spent some time warming her up – first we showered together, then a massage, then kissing and nibbling. She started panting, moaning and writhing around, getting more and more excited at my touch, I did not stop. I slowly started caressing her pussy – eventually inserting two fingers and rubbing the G-spot.

When she said she had to urinate, she seemed uncomfortable and wanted to stop. However, I would not quit toying with the G-Spot. She almost forced me off her, but then the sensation kicked in! She not only had one G-gasm, she had four! The rate and the frequency of G-gasms increase with each love making session. The most she has ever had in one night has been 17, which is so incredible!

Every chance I get, I spread the word about the G-gasm Method. I only hope it helps people as much as it has helped us."

Ann Marie S.

RE: "WOW, THIS IS BETTER THAN FUN!"

Ann Marie, that is awesome. I think that the sensation of having to pee is the number one reason some couples have trouble experiencing G-gasms. Once she gets past that hurdle – it is ecstasy! Good work BTW with the not quitting.

"TRIED IT ... LOVED IT"

"I knew from the moment I found out about the Method that I wanted to try it. However, as a single woman I did not know when I would be able to try it out. I tried with my own fingers but the positioning made it hard to reach. I decided to buy a G-Spot vibrator and had excellent results with that, but obviously, that is only a close second to a warm body. There is a big difference between a woman making love to you and a vibrator giving you massive G-gasms – although the vibrator is highly pleasurable.

I am writing this today because I finally got a chance to experience it first hand (LOL). Wow! I never imagined anything so fulfilling! I was lucky enough to meet someone that actually knew the Method, and laughed when I told her that I wanted to try it. She tied me down so that I could not get away and spent the entire evening exploring my body. I had 25 G-gasms from G-Spot manipulation alone! This is not including the other orgasms I had that night.

This is fabulous! I do not know how I used to live with only one orgasm!"

Cathy L.

RE: "TRIED IT ... LOVED IT"

Cathy – It is tough for you to succeed with the Method with your own fingers. You can reach the G-spot OK, but most girls cannot stroke with enough pressure to G-gasm. To increase the pressure, with two fingers in your pussy place the palm of your other hand on your abdomen right above your pubic bone - just below your navel and squeeze down with your palm, while pressing up and out with your fingers.

Great selection of toys at: g-gasm.com/toys

Glad to see you found a FWB.

"DISAPPOINTED"

"I have only tried this once but I have to voice my disappointment. Although we followed the steps properly, the Method did not work. We tried it while I was lying on my stomach and then on my back. We even tried it on my side. My partner tried soft and hard rubbing and though it felt good for a brief amount of time, I never got past the urination feeling.

I have never had any nerve damage or anything so I am not sure why this problem is occurring. We do know that he hit the G-Spot- any advise."

Shawnee

RE: "DISAPPOINTED"

Man, do you give up easy! You tried it all of one time and you're done. You'll be sorry … No, seriously don't give up yet.

I am guessing it has to do with poor muscle control. Forget about the Method for a few weeks. Start doing some Kegel exercises to strengthen you PC muscles – we talked about that in the book – this will help you get past that "I have to pee and am not comfortable" hurdle.

What is your lover's email address – I want to send her a note to tell her to make you as HORNY AS FUCKING POSSIBLE before she goes poking around the G-spot. This is especially important the first few times you try the G-gasm Method.

"HOW LONG SHOULD I RUB"

"Thank you for this great information. Last night, my lady and I were experimenting with the G-gasm Method. She claims that she has a big butt, (I love it just the way it is) so is a bit uncomfortable laying face down, with her ass up in the air. She propped herself up on one knee – almost at a 45 degree angle from her hips to bed. She lifted her leg a bit, and I inserted my thumb from behind.

She was hot, and came within 30 seconds. I kept rubbing, and she kept moaning as if she was constantly cumming for about 5 minutes. Eventually she went limp – I actually had to check if she was still breathing.

My question is – when should I stop rubbing? Thanks."

Rita the limo driver

RE: "HOW LONG SHOULD I RUB"

Hey Rita –

Glad to see you gals having fun. I like to keep the G-gasms going in a rolling pattern. Build her up to a G-gasm, stop rubbing for a few seconds to a minute, and then start rubbing again. This gives her a little break, but not enough of a breather to let her down from her sexual high.

If she is in shape physically, you can keep her cumming for hours or until you get a thumb cramp (which you will get until you build up your thumb muscles). Mix it up a little – give her one huge 5 minute G-gasm, then add some mini G-gasms followed by a mother lode G-gasm, followed by some edging (bringing her to the brink of a G-gasm, but then stop rubbing thereby putting off the G-gasm), followed by the mother of all G-gasms. The power is all yours Rita.

Vary it up, add some toys, add some spankings (if she's been a bad girl) – try it different times of day or night. Your lady will appreciate your dedication to **her** pleasure.

"SHOCKING!"

"First off, let me start by saying that I do not know how to thank you enough. This Method has changed my life. My sex life was good before, but this is just ridiculous. We use the Method regularly and in many different positions. After she warms me up with her magic fingers, I get off by her doing me doggy style. Fun! This Method has turned me into a nymphomaniac for sure LOL.

The sensations are incredibly hard to describe. The feelings stretch from my toes all the way to the top of my head. My body tingles and I explode in pleasure. Once the first G-gasm hits, I am lost in the sensations. I reach at least 20 G-gasms per night, but have had many more when we have longer love sessions. I have had a chance to use this with more than one sex partner and it works with all of them – I leave your book lying around the living room table. Only problem is that some girls are harder to train than others are :o).

Thank you for sharing such a wonderful Method with the world. Now that I have learned how to master it I seriously could not imagine living without this pleasure in my life!"

RE: "SHOCKING ORGASMS!"

You are most welcome! When can I come over for "training?"

"I'M TRYING!"

"My girlfriend found out about your Method from some friends and could not wait to try it. I had no problem because I love to give her pleasure but our results are not as successful as I could have hoped. There was literally no sensation for her when it came to this activity. I tried for some time, but no reaction from her. She didn't even get to the needing to pee feeling. I wanted to be able to wow her with this but unfortunately I think I am one of the small percentages of women that just do not know what they are doing."

RE: "I'M TRYING!"

Keep at it, don't ever give up. Remember, that all women are different. Some take a little longer to wake up the G-spot – but once it is awake – WATCH OUT! Do not make this out to be some kind of an experiment – weave the Method into your other sexual activities. You are not baking a cake; do not tell her you are going to try "something new." Don't act like a gynecologist, act like a lover as you make love to her G-spot.

Take your time making love to her. What is her "hot spot?" Does she like oral stimulation? If so, get her to the brink of a clit orgasm a few times. Do not let her cum; just get her close to climax. Get her a hot as fucking possible without her going over the edge.

When you see she is really starting to boil over, get

her comfortable and face down over some pillows. Kiss her back, nibble her ass – you know, all the stuff you normally do – you do normally do that … right? Get her to relax and gently work your thumb into her now drenching wet pussy. Star rubbing slowly and softly, as she gets more excited, increase the pressure and speed of your rubbing. She has to get used to the new thing that your thumb is doing. It does feel weird for her the first time; get her to relax and build her up slowly.

Once she G-gasms the first time, get rougher with the G-spot to keep her cumming for a long time.

"WOW"

"This was amazing. I am multi-orgasmic as it is, and it really doesn't take much to bring me to an orgasmic state. When my lady brought this information to me, we were interested in trying this to see how it would work for us. Things did work well. In fact, I will admit I had at least 20 orgasms that night in a span of the two hours we were messing around.

I pass it on whenever I can. I know many of my female friends are impressed with the results. If the women were multi-orgasmic they state that it feels great, but they are not quite as amazed as the women that were used to only one orgasm per evening."

RE: "WOW"

Being naturally multi-orgasmic gives you a head start on the one O per night girls --- but they will catch up! Enjoy!

"TWO G-SPOTS ARE MORE FUN THAN ONE"

"My girlfriend bought your book. We both read it, I have to admit I was a bit skeptical, but we decided to try it. What happened next is something I will never forget. It took us a couple of times to perfect the Method but it works well on both of us. Not only does one of us benefit with this Method we both do! We managed to work out a situation where we can have G-gasms together using either our fingers on each other or using a double-ended dildo.

This was the best thing that has ever happened to us. What is even more amazing is that before this I swore the G-Spot did not even exist. Neither of us had the pleasure of experiencing anything like it. Thank you so much for sharing this excellent information."

Shawna and Robbee

RE: "TWO G-SPOTS ARE MORE ... "

Oh my gosh ... is it getting hot in here? Can someone please open a window!

"STILL WORKING AT IT"

"It has been fun and exciting for me. At times, frustrating but you know what they say ... practice makes perfect. Since my girlfriend has started reading your book, she has become much more open about her feelings, especially during our love making sessions.

Thank you for the advice, we have both learned a great deal about our bodies and ourselves. Trust is not an issue – we have been together over 20 years and we spend

90% of our free time together.

I think there are some ingrained inhibitions floating around. We are working on them but still it has been a very pleasurable journey for the both of us. We haven't gone to the bank with any G-gasms yet, but you have revitalized our marriage and made us feel like stupid teenagers again just discovering sex.

WTF – I thought I knew everything! You rock – thanks."

Kelly

Kelly – Often I think of my own upbringing. My parents would never dream of discussing sex never mind female/female relationships. There is no wonder that people have inhibitions hovering around the cobwebs of the mind. Did you or your lady have a religious upbringing? Think of all the nonsense they teach there. These thoughts go back in your psyche and couples sometimes need professional help – I always use my local bartender – he makes me feel better about myself … at least for a little while.

Good luck … let me know how you make out. At least I turned you into horny fucking teenagers again.

"WHO KNEW?"

"I cannot thank you enough! I have never had a very fulfilling sex life but my girlfriend is a miracle worker when it comes to perfecting this Method. She has always been very patient and caring about my needs. She sprung this on me on a Sunday afternoon; I was in complete shock with what happened. She asked me to trust her, but I was nervous when she began holding me down.

At first it might seemed a little intense -- with the "have to pee" feeling, but I worked through it. The sensations are so worth it, I can't even begin to explain. The first G-gasm hit me like a ton of bricks. She let up for a few seconds then attacked my G- spot harder and faster; I came so fast and so powerfully that I think I literary arched into the air. It was beautiful - total mayhem. She played with different angles with her two fingers, rubbing in all sorts of motions, teasing me, working me into a G-gasm, then stopping and making me beg. My current record is set at 15! Thank you so much for sharing this wonderful knowledge with the world.

When someone peels me off the ceiling, I want to buy you dinner."

RE: "WHO KNEW?"

Awesome ... let me know when you get up to 50 per night.

"CAN'T GET ENOUGH"

"I have told everyone I know about this fabulous Method. I tried it out the day I found out about it and have used it regularly since then. You are simply fabulous for sharing this information because women all over the world are now able to experience what they should have been experiencing all along.

We both recently turned 18 and got our own place, my girlfriend and I have never been more satisfied. She walks around all day glowing because she is so happy and relaxed. We are able to do this in multiple positions and with different angles. Each one makes her scream in a different way. We have not had this much sex since we were teenagers. Again, thank you so much. This is just great."

RE: "CAN'T GET ENOUGH"

Ahhh … to be 18 again. I don't know if my body could take it … do I get a fresh liver to replace the one in the wagon? Enjoy!

"NEW SEX POSITION"

"Last night, I was on my hands and knees, my girlfriend behind me, he inserted one finger, then a second finger in my pussy. This really got the juices flowing, but then he put his thumb in my butt. He was opening and closing his fingers and thumb like a mouth. I was shaking … the bed was soaked ... he said he could feel it running over the back of his hand."

Maggie K.

RE: "SEX POSITION"

That's the beauty of the Method – there is no right or wrong way to perform. Do and try anything that intensifies the feelings – the more things you add to the mix the better.

I've tried dildos, extra fingers, two thumbs, veggies, tongue, talking dirty, nipple clamps, paddles (... that wonderful line between pleasure and pain), restraints, porn – you name it … I'll try it at least twice to make sure it's right. Just when I think I have reached the limit – I find a new ingredient.

My favorite position is lady face down, butt up in the air, insert thumb, rub and wait for the pyrotechnics to start. The great thing about using the thumb is that it keeps you from targeting too deep in the pussy and you can get a good hard rub going.

AUTOGASMS

Many women have written in to talk about something amazing called an autogasm. The autogasm is a new phenomenon that occurs when the body is in a blissful state from receiving so much pleasure. Mini G-gasms continue for hours after any sexual activity has ended. A woman that is able to have them will never forget them.

I have never been with a woman that has experienced autogasms, but from talking to couples that have had the pleasure, they are a series of mini G-gasms that recur as the lady is coming down from her sexual high. In all cases, the love making sessions were long and intense, lasting more than two hours with the lady experiencing 20 or more G-gasms in that period.

Again, not all couples encounter autogasms. Imagine your lady going to work after a 20 something G-gasm session.

"Roche, why are you walking so funny?" asked Mr. Klumpkin, her boss at work.

"Oh, I don't know ... Karen and I were ... oh my gosh ... what the fuck ... oh man ... no way ... this is not ... oh gooooowwddd ...."

"Roche, what's the matter? Can I get you some water?"

"Towel … please …"

GALS ... A WARNING!

This is a very powerful Method. You are the giver of great pleasure. Your lover may not being able to think about anything else but being in your bed ... you could call it obsessed.

The most important thing you need to remember is that every woman's body is different. The standard Method will not work on all women, which is why I provide multiple options and variations. One variation may work, while others will not. However, if you are showing them the time and attention they need they will often have a great time regardless of whether it works fully or not. There is no such thing as 'bad sex.'

Don't take this knowledge too technically and never treat the event as a "sex workshop" about being able to make a woman have that many orgasms. All that does is make it harder on you and less enjoyable for her. This is all about pleasing her.

I received this e-mail from one of my readers Cindy S.

"My girlfriend Linda and I love your book – I'm perfectly happy stimulating her to the point of G-Gasm after G-Gasm. Our sex life has never been better.

The other day, I went on our computer, there was an open window with Google search results – the phrase Linda was searching for – "how to please my woman."

Thanks!

Cindy S."

As a willing partner, you will get yours. Trust me, she will want to please you as much as you satisfied her. You are going to hear this:

"How the hell did you do that?"

You are entering a completely new paradigm regarding sex – a new way of performing and pleasing your partner. More than likely, you will be introducing her to her G-spot. She may have read about it, heard about it or maybe even played with her G-spot; what you are going to introduce, she has never experienced sexually. It is a complete change in consciousness, a new approach to sex.

You will reach a higher level of connection with your lover when she trusts you enough to let go. Jena described it to me as, "What a woman feels with the Method is hard to explain with words, unless you have experienced it, there is no way you can understand. Once you get past, the urge to pee you have broken through the last obstruction and given yourself entirely to your partner, who now must have your total trust. The lack of trust is a reason that some women do not experience G-gasms the way they should.

Many-experienced woman find this Method scary or uncomfortable. They have been used to controlling the destiny of their orgasms, and now they cannot – you are in charge.

Definitely, take it slow with a sexually inexperienced lady. Could you imagine, a girl that has been playing around with masturbation and here you come along and blow her away with 20 or 30 dripping wet, massive G-gasms. Take it easy, take it slow, do the stuff you should be doing first like necking, heavy petting before you start with G-gasms.

What exactly does this mean? This means, that this Method is all about pleasing her. She has to trust you enough to hand over the controls to her body, because she will be helpless once the G-gasms start. She must let go completely. She will be screaming "OH MY GOSH" until her throat is sore and eyes rolling back in her head. There is nothing ladylike about it. The first time, she could actually get scared.

If she is used to gentle rubbing and stroking, she will find that the G-gasm Method is much more intense and physical than a clitoral orgasm. Oral sex for a woman is usually the best. Now you have something better in your arsenal. You can literally keep her going for hours until she hyperventilates or passes out. She will be thrashing and screaming.

The best part is afterwards, she will be glowing like a hot light bulb in a cold hard steel pot. Her self confidence will be at an all time high. Many women need that "loving" thing at the end of a G-gasm session, so they don't feel like they are being used or abused. They need to re-establish intimate contact and connect with you, kind of like being welcomed back from a long trip. Many soft kisses, embracing, caressing, you know - mushy stuff - that some girlfriends crave. Describe to her how incredibly fucking sexy and turned on you were, by watching her cum like that. She will feel even better knowing that you had a good time too.

You on the other hand, will be strutting around the room like a well-oiled sex god. You will feel like you are ten feet tall because of what you did to her. Any kind of sex related problems you thought you had are now gone.

You get a tremendous sense of satisfaction knowing you have given your woman THAT much pleasure. It is incredible. It also gives you a feeling of confidence whenever you look at a woman and knowing what you could do for her.

Gals, you will know why it truly is better to give than to receive. The look on her face is priceless. There is nothing more satisfying than hearing her scream with pleasure, teasing her, and knowing that she is getting off because of you. Use this outline of the G-gasm Method as a roadmap to pleasure, but sometimes the most enjoyable parts are the detours.

This is an incredible Method to master, something you and your lover have to work on, to make her a multi-orgasmic, quivering, sweaty, sticky, convulsing, twitching mess every time you make love. Completely awesome. Enjoy!

APPENDIX A – EXERCISE

HAND

Your only concern now is the condition of your hands and fingers. The last thing you want to do is to have an awesome G-gasm session going on and before she can scream UNCLE, your hand cramps up. That's not good. Let's say you only gave her about only ten G-gasms and she wants and needs 30 or more. If your hand craps out, she is going to be pissed.

First thing to remember is that most everyone has two hands and ten fingers. If your right thumb is getting tired, switch to your left hand, if your thumb is getting cramped flip her over and use your fingers.

I have found that the thumb can last longer than fingers doing the "come here" motion. The thumb is in a direct line with the larger arm and shoulder muscles. With the "come here" motion, all the movement is with your hand muscles; using your thumb, you use your thumb muscle, arm muscles and shoulder muscles.

Squeezing a hard rubber ball is a good method of hand exercise. If you want to spend a few bucks, get some handgrips with added weights. Start with small sets of squeezing, and work your way up to 100 hundred or more.

PC MUSCLES – KEGELS FOR LADIES

Kegel exercises created originally to help women strengthen their PC muscles to help stop urinary incontinence after childbirth. The Kegel exercise turns out, has sexual benefits also.

Ladies, there are three reasons you should do your Kegel exercises.

First, a strong PC muscle will help you overcome the "have to pee" feeling during the G-gasm Method.

Second, with the PC muscle stretched out, less of the vagina and G-spot area are in direct contact with the fingers or dildo and therefore receives less stimulation – less fun for you and your partner.

Thirdly, a well-toned PC muscle will give you a powerful ejaculation. Keep the PC muscle exercised with Kegels – you will have greater blood flow to this area, and the greater ability to become aroused and feel sexual pleasure.

The great thing about doing Kegel exercises is that no one knows you are doing them. While you can do all sorts of variations, the basic Kegel exercises are:

Contract your PC muscles. Hold initially for a count of five; build up gradually to a count of twenty. Repeat ten times and practice daily. Like with all muscles you are better off building the PC muscle slowly and regularly.

You can also add quick Kegels, contracting and releasing the muscle for ten seconds. Relax for a few moments and then do it again. Try a "rolling" Kegel with your PC muscle, squeeze only at the entrance to your vagina initially, and then rolling the contraction up the length of your vagina and back down.

Spread the word – let the G-gasms roll!

Please visit us online at g-gasm.com

www.ingramcontent.com/pod-product-compliance
Ingram Content Group UK Ltd.
Pitfield, Milton Keynes, MK11 3LW, UK
UKHW041412180426
11947UKWH00007B/83